Power and Praise

Navigating life
from a higher perspective

DR AFINIKI AKANET

Power and Praise
by Afiniki Akanet

Produced and published in 2024
by Affinity Global Enterprises (AGE) Ltd
www.afiniki.co.uk

Paperback ISBN: 978-1-7397416-3-1
Ebook ISBN: 978-1-7397416-4-8

Dedication

To everyone who wants to live an extraordinary life

Glory belongs to God, whose power is at work in us. By this power He can do infinitely more than we can ask or imagine. Glory belongs to God in the church and in Christ Jesus for all time and eternity! Amen - Ephesians 3:20-21

Did you know that "spirituality and religion:

- Promote a positive worldview
- Help to make sense of difficult situations
- Give purpose and meaning
- Discourage maladaptive coping
- Enhance social support
- Promote 'other-directedness'
- Help to release the need for control
- Provide and encourage forgiveness
- Encourage thankfulness
- Provide hope"?

Spirituality in Psychiatry,
Andrew Sims and Christopher C. H. Cook,
Royal College of Psychiatry Publications

"Mental health is critically important for everyone, everywhere, and goes beyond the mere absence of a mental health condition. It is integral to well-being, enabling people to realise their full potential, show resilience amidst adversity, be productive across the various settings of daily life, form meaningful relationships and contribute to their communities. Physical, psychological, social, cultural, **spiritual** and other interrelated factors contribute to mental health, and there are inseparable links between mental and physical health."

- World Health Organisation

Reviews of Power and Praise:

"A supremely practical and useful book. Original, palatable, and honest advice based on lived experiences, by a trained professional" - Arup Roy, Lead Surface Design Engineer

"Niki writes in a lovely conversational style that makes it sound like a conversation with a friend. The book offers insight into the worldview of the author and how it shapes even the smallest decisions and experiences in her life. It challenges the reader to view life from a different perspective and encourages reflection on what is important. It is hopeful and encouraging in its tone. Power and Praise *is worth a read."* - Zainab Oseni, General Practitioner (GP) with a special interest in global health

"In this book, Niki gives so many anecdotes of situations/problems she has encountered in her life, followed by extremely helpful suggestions of how she overcame them...Niki is such a prolific writer that once you start reading this or any of her other books, they are hard to put down until you reach the end. I highly recommend this book." - Margaret Greenway, Retired administrator

Other books by Dr Afiniki Akanet

All available from Afiniki.co.uk and Amazon.co.uk

- Fortitude (The Story of a Nigerian Girl in the UK)
- Felicity
- Life Without Coffee (Choosing Happiness Over Stress)
- Taking CSA Tomorrow (Get in the right mindset for your MRCGP exam)
- 2020, Year of Plenty
- Money and Mental Wellbeing

To find out more about the author: Afiniki.co.uk

For inspirational gifts and items: MyLivingHope.co.uk

CONTENTS

Introduction

Thank you for choosing this book, even with such a broad title, *Power and Praise*, which I look forward to unpacking with you. I decided to write this book in the year that I turn 40, as a representation of my gratitude for life and as my reflection on the experiences of my first four decades on earth. You could also consider it a continuation of the mission accomplished through my previous books, *Life Without Coffee (Choosing Happiness Over Stress)* and *Money and Mental Wellbeing*, which have served as self-help resources for improving mental health for people around the world.

The four years before my 40th birthday have been very interesting, with working through the COVID-19 pandemic as a UK General Practitioner (GP/family doctor) and joining a GP partnership (co-owning a GP surgery) in 2022. So many lives were lost and changed during the pandemic, so I do not take it for granted to be alive and well after all we went through, especially as frontline healthcare workers. My thoughts are with the families of those who lost loved ones, and people still struggling with the effects of long covid. Life is full of ups and downs, which is why we have each other to lean on, and why I am so passionate about sharing ideas that help us to overcome life's challenges.

It was great to have the opportunity to become a GP partner in 2022, because I was working in my first salaried GP role, not planning to become a GP partner for another three years, at least. I decided to do my junior doctor training for General Practice part-time while having our two children, after a financially and mentally challenging journey to getting my medical degree. I felt so happy to finally be doing what I love and did not mind that I was a 'mature student' at medical school and older than many newly qualified GPs. The long journey to becoming a doctor actually helped me to build resilience, faith and inner strength, to become an author and start an educational charity, Forte Charity for Inspiration, which celebrated 15 years of existence in 2023. Truly, "all things work together for good for those who love God and are called according to His purpose" (Romans 8:28).

In 2022, I was preparing to travel to Abidjan (Ivory Coast) to do some work with Forte Charity, so I used one of my days off work to attend the interview, where I met my lovely business partners. There was an instant connection, and on my request, they were willing to offer me a partnership position, instead of the usual 'salaried-with-a-view-to-partnership' deal. Most GPs try out a workplace for at least a few months before committing to becoming a partner there, and we have always been advised to be very careful about getting into partnerships because the commitment can be as serious as marriage in many ways. I never worked a day at my surgery before taking on the GP partnership post, and thankfully, I still have no regrets about this decision.

I do not take my commitments to marriage and partnership lightly - I am also celebrating 14 years of marriage in the year that I turn 40, and am so grateful to God for the great relationship I still have with my loving husband. My friend used to say that we can only confirm if we made good marriage decisions if we are still happy together after 10, 20 or 30 years because a great wedding and honeymoon mean nothing in the grand scheme of things. I think she was right, and I am very grateful to have a supportive life partner to go into the next phase of life with. People say that "Life begins at 40", so I am excited to see all that the future holds for us. I am nowhere near where I used to be but am also not yet where I want to be, so I look forward with hope for a brighter future. When I joined my GP surgery as the youngest partner, I took a personality test, which we offer to all staff. I was excited to see that my personality animal was an eagle. I remember the senior partner commenting that I was the "only air-borne member of the management team". It reminded me so much of this Bible verse, which still strengthens me today as I try to live life from a higher viewpoint:

But those who trust in the Lord will find new strength. They will soar high on wings like eagles. They will run and not grow weary. They will walk and not faint - Isaiah 40:31

Spirituality is now recognised as an important part of our existence, which is connected to our physical and mental health. A Spirituality and Psychiatry Special Interest Group (SPSIG) was founded in 1999 within the Royal College of Psychiatrists

(RCPsych) to increase knowledge of the research linking spirituality with health and raise the profile of spirituality in patient care. Even so, this remains the aspect least researched and discussed in healthcare settings, which is why I will be touching more on my spirituality and how it connects to mental health in this book. Spirituality has been described as a sense of seeking the best relationship with ourselves, others and what may lie 'beyond' to help us have meaning, purpose, hope and support even in times of loss and suffering, which we all face at some point in our lives. Spirituality can be seen as a beautiful journey, but can sadly also be seen as stressful and unattractive when negative experiences and unhelpful practices are involved. In this book, I will be sharing thoughts and practices that have helped me to look after my spiritual and mental health.

Spirituality is not about being religious, because we know that spirituality is more than simply belonging to a religion. It is more about how we see our place in the world and the meaning we give to the events of our lives. Dr Nick Hallett shared a great example of why we need to understand spirituality when talking about mental health in his Royal College of Psychiatry publication, *Why Spirituality Matters in Psychiatry.* He described seeing a mentally unwell woman who was very distressed with disordered thoughts and self-neglect. She was behaving in a chaotic way, which was out of character for her, and kept leaving her house at night with bags packed because she believed Jesus Christ would come back imminently and she needed to find where He would return. She could not explain on what basis she knew Jesus would return that night and denied any possibility that she could be mistaken. Within the context of her presentation, she was deemed to have a delusional conviction, which mentally unwell patients can have. I remember being surprised at how many unwell patients had beliefs related to religion/spirituality when I worked in psychiatry myself.

Dr Nick Hallett explained that he later found out that her very concerned family also believed in the future return of Jesus Christ - but at an unknown time, which was consistent with their Christian beliefs. They knew that others might not share their beliefs and had thought processes consistent with "normal" religious beliefs that were not delusional. He concluded that best practice for doctors requires an understanding of normal spiritual/religious beliefs and practices to be able to distinguish them from mental illness so that people are not mislabeled for having normal human experiences. Everyone, notwithstanding their mental state, will have to face the important questions of meaning, identity and purpose at some point in life, and this is another reason why spirituality is relevant for everyone - patients and professionals alike. He concluded that "Practising psychiatry without understanding or addressing spiritual issues cannot be good psychiatry from the perspective of either clinician or patient. As mental health becomes increasingly acknowledged in the media and society, the need for understanding and addressing our patients' spiritual issues is too important to ignore."

For me, life has been an exciting journey of growth and discovery, which has been so much sweeter because of the amazing people in my life, who are just too many to mention. I believe that the most important reason I have for feeling spiritually healthy, with joy and peace in my life is the fact that I made a very important decision many years ago in Sunday

School to put my faith in Jesus, which is a decision people make every day all around the world. I must have been five or six years old then in Nigeria, but that is a decision that shaped my future decisions to build the life I now enjoy. Interestingly, it was also around that time that I told my parents that I wanted to become a medical doctor. The peace and joy I experience from having Jesus as my God and His Holy Spirit as my guide cannot be completely expressed in words. God cares about every aspect of our lives, even career and marriage decisions! I learned and believed that I cannot save myself from the natural sinful nature we all have which separates us from God who is so holy, but sent His perfect only Son (Jesus) to pay for the sins (wrong-doing) of the world (including me), so that anyone who believes in Jesus (accepting that His death and resurrection has paid the price for us to have a relationship with God and gain eternal life in heaven) will enjoy abundant life, joy and peace as a child of God. I am so grateful to be a child of God, through faith in Jesus, the only wise God, who works all things together for good. His arms are still wide open for all who will believe in Him, accept His love and surrender to His great plan for their lives. This is a choice I have made for my life, and I appreciate that others might choose a different path, so I hope that whatever spiritual path you choose, you can apply some principles shared from this book to help you enjoy life.

I experienced intense grief after suddenly losing a very close family friend in July 2023. I remember weeping uncontrollably at work with the burden of grief, that I had to be comforted by nurses and sent home by my supportive partners. That was a real humble pie moment for someone like me who wants to be strong and there to look after everyone else.

Even though we never stop missing people we love after they are gone, we can draw strength from the fact that they would want us to keep on living. I have since experienced divine comfort and can look back on happy memories of him with a smile, even through tears, knowing that we will meet again in heaven. We also had some difficult health challenges in my family in 2023, as many others have and may still sadly be having, but I am so grateful that it has all ended in praise and thanksgiving. Happiness usually depends on what is happening in our lives, but the joy and peace that Jesus gives me cannot be destroyed, even in the face of pain, cancer and death. There is so much more to say, but I have decided to keep this book short. I cannot finish this section without saying a very special thank you to the two people who have been there for me since my birthday in 1984 and have been wonderful parents to me - thank you so much, Mum and Dad (Grace and Iliya Akanet)! Having children of my own has helped me to truly appreciate my parents and all that they did, and still do, to help me become the woman I am today. I will not hear the end of it if I do not mention my favourite children - Sophie and David, who love reading and make me a very happy mum! Now, let's talk about power and praise...

CHAPTER 1
What We Want

The age-old question

There are so many ideas about what humans want most in life. Some talk about love, attention and understanding. Others mention safety, belonging and achievement. Others say it is social acceptance and respect. A popular one is power (control), attraction (connection), comfort (safety) and play (freedom). We are told the basic need for survival (food, water, shelter, safety) is accompanied by primal desires for companionship and reproduction. It is indeed a complex answer, especially as times move on and people find it more difficult to know and express what they really want. The expression of such desires becomes even more complex when we consider how this affects others in a free world. We hear on the news how one person's desire for a different gender or sexual satisfaction can lead to offence or the abuse of others; how someone's desire for control/power can fuel betrayal, dictatorship and wars; and how someone's desire for more money and comfort can lead to poverty and stress for others. People casually mention "world peace" and "love" when asked what they want, but what does it take to achieve this?

In my experience, most people just want to be happy. What it takes to make them happy is a different matter. I have a staff wellbeing role in my GP job and also as a school governor, and the staff wellbeing surveys we usually take show that happiness is often related to people's expectations and perceptions of change. Some people will be happy no matter what, and others will always have a reason to complain. In a work context, we have to consider that there are home issues and personal factors influencing people's levels of happiness, but we keep doing our best to ensure that everyone can have job satisfaction because we know that happy employees are more productive. When there is a good atmosphere at work, with everyone feeling valued and safe, people are happy to be there. I think that *peace* is what people really want because no one wants to spend eight to twelve hours of their day with constant criticism, stress and anxiety. When we feel psychologically safe, we can think more clearly to come up with better ideas and solutions to problems, which will lead to happier, productive lives.

It is difficult, even in a home environment for people to thrive if there is no peace. Chaos and anxiety at home can make children struggle to learn and succeed. Relationship problems can make people struggle to concentrate/succeed in work and business. There is little chance of economic or personal progress in a war-torn area, with displaced citizens and hurt people. An atmosphere of peace in and around us gives us the power to think more clearly and achieve the goals that make us happy while considering the impact of our decisions on others in a less selfish manner. People who perpetrate evil and injustice are not people of peace, which is why they try to find happiness by hurting others. Because power and control are considered to be common human desires, we should prioritise our need for peace of mind and peaceful relationships with others so that we can retain the power to prosper. Peace of mind is priceless, especially when we realise the power it holds to help us find true happiness.

Pursue peace

Realising the power that peace brings encourages me to maintain peace in my life. If we are not intentional about this, we can easily find ourselves in difficult situations that could have been avoided. I am particularly keen on maintaining peace in my home because that is where I spend most of my time and that is where my children live. I know that a peaceful atmosphere at home helps them feel secure and confident to face the world and any challenges that may come their way. I, myself, am also less productive in a chaotic environment, so I protect my peace as a way of guarding my productivity and purpose. A peaceful home is not just about order and silence, but love and harmony. I learned years ago that stress and disputes make me less likely to have good ideas for writing, work and business, so I continue to choose happiness over stress through the wisdom that God gives. There may be a lot of problems around me, but if my heart is at peace, there is really no stress. My happiness also leads to having a happier marriage and a successful husband who can support me. We all need to take responsibility for our own happiness, rather than giving such a heavy burden to a spouse or anyone else.

As they say, a happy marriage is made up of two good forgivers. We forgive not because people deserve it, but because we deserve peace. When two people manage their emotions well, the relationship can move forward with less drama. We thrash out issues between us promptly to avoid bad weeks that might lead to bad months and a bad life. I remember talking some time ago with my husband about the need to "fight for peace". Some people think that peace is about sweeping issues under the carpet and pretending that everything is okay to avoid confronting important issues. I have tried that before and it doesn't work. What happens when we do that is that the issues pile up, we become bitter without inner peace and start to act out in unusual ways, which may not be helpful for the relationship. This is often the weak point when people become vulnerable to negative outside influences and mental illness that might end up breaking up the relationship/marriage. When we truly understand the negative impact of divorce on our mental health and children, maintaining peace in our marriages will become a top priority.

Maintaining peace in our lives, homes and workplaces is not about the things we do once in a while. It is mostly about the things we do every day, the habits and routines we have that make people feel loved, wanted and respected. This is where intentional living comes in. When we choose to work late every night, we are choosing to spend less time with family and choosing to create a culture at work that may be impacting the mental health of staff negatively. When we choose to kiss our family good night/morning every day, no matter what, we are choosing to maintain contact and provide reassurance even when we have had a disagreement. When we choose to eat dinner together regularly as a family, we are intentionally providing daily opportunities for people to talk, not just when things go wrong. When we check on and laugh with our staff regularly (not only when there is a complaint or a party), we are choosing to keep communication lines open for a happier workplace. When we choose to pray daily, not only when we are in trouble, we are also choosing to depend on God (not our human strength) for the future.

I have learned not to complain about things I tolerate. If something bothers me that much, I do something about it. I believe in God as my heavenly Father who is caring and All-Powerful. Over the years, I have pursued peace at home and work by praying about issues, facing difficult conversations and making necessary changes, which were not always easy. The peace of God gives me clarity to receive guidance from His Holy Spirit when I pray according to God's will. We can choose to believe and speak what God says in His Word (the Holy Bible) rather than the negative things we see, because the Bible says that "we walk by faith and not by sight" (2 Corinthians 5:7). Even when things are tough, we can acknowledge and empathise, but be careful not dwell in the pit of pity, because "God has not given us a spirit of fear, but of power, of love and a sound mind" (2 Timothy 1:7). Holding on to that peace, helps me to maintain a sound mind and keep the power we have as children of God.

Life is short

People are quick to say that life is short and we must have fun, but I think of life being "short" as a reason to use time wisely and leave a good legacy. If it all boils down to a hyphen, I want the hyphen between 1984 and whatever year Jesus takes me to heaven to be significant when it is put on my grave. I want to use all the talents, opportunities and skills that God has given me for good. I want to share and write what I can to make the world a better place. I want to be the reason that people say "Thank God!" because their prayers have been answered by God's power working through me. I want my whole life and work to be an expression of the goodness of our wonderful Maker. Having this perspective brings me to the realisation that time is precious and there is still so much to be done.

All this does not happen by chance. I have to intentionally put aside my selfish desires for God's will to be done through me, if I want to see the full manifestation of His will for my life. It can be hard to be patient when things in life are not happening as quickly as I would want. It can be tough being different or working differently from others, but I am blessed because so many experiences from my past have helped me to get comfortable with standing out. We can sometimes get tempted to do things our way and forget about godly principles. It can even be hard to humble ourselves or give up our time to do the kinds of things God asks of us, as part of His great plan, which we usually have only a tiny glimpse of, but there is always a joy that comes with total obedience. The hard part is that, as Christians, we also are not to do things for praise or recognition, but to please our heavenly Father. Our good deeds may end up bringing us those things, but that should not be the motive for doing what we do, which is why we do not broadcast every good work we do. There is greatness in us all, but we see throughout history that those who become truly great were not pursuing greatness after all. Jesus says in the Bible that the greatest in His kingdom is the servant of all. This is a big mystery that we only grasp by His grace. When we acknowledge our weaknesses and realise that His grace is sufficient for us, we can go out boldly into the world, knowing that our power comes from Almighty God who cannot be defeated.

I have found that the more I know God, the more confident I am to be and do all He wants me to. This is why I consider it an excellent use of my time to study His Word, the Holy Bible, and listen to teachings/podcasts about growing in Christ. You might know Christians who are full of flaws and foolishness, making you wonder whether they follow the same Jesus I am referring to. I also have flaws and have not reached full maturity in Christ, but that does not mean that His power in us is any less potent. It is up to us, even after we have put our faith in Jesus, to open our minds to the renewal He promises through His Word, so that our lives are transformed, powerful and Christ-like to make a greater impact in the world around us. Someone once said that, as Christians, God should be "present, obvious and powerful" in *every* area of our lives. I liked that it made me think of God P.O.Ping through us.

If we stay focused on the mistakes of the past, we cannot move on to leave a great legacy. Peter, who denied Jesus three times, as recorded in the Bible, ended up doing great miracles and good works after he repented. But Judas, who betrayed Jesus and could not see past his sin, ended up hanging himself and becoming an example of how Satan destroys lives. Every day is a chance to start afresh and do better by the power of God which is available to us through faith and prayer. We can then look back and see how far we have come, but keep growing intentionally while we still have life. After all is said and done, I want to have lived a life worthy of emulation and enjoy eternity in heaven. I am so grateful that every day is an opportunity to do better.

Leading from the back

It is true that not everyone wants to be a boss or leader at the front. Not everyone wants to be wealthy or "great" as the world sees it. Some people are happier with less responsibility and attention. We are all made differently for a reason. If everyone leads from the front, there will be no one to follow. Leaders need people to support them and help make things happen. Some people feel so uncomfortable with praise and commendation but are quick to encourage and compliment others. They are confident in their supporting roles and do it to the best of their ability with joy. When we realise that greatness is not about standing in front or being boss, we can appreciate the part that everyone plays in making the world a better place. Even great leaders have to follow at times. Life is in seasons. We learn to be in authority by being under authority. No matter how high you go in life, you will find that there is always someone to answer to.

The sooner we learn to respect and appreciate authority, the better it will be for our growth journey. The first authority in my life is God, who gives me life and hope. He has also given me a husband to be the head of my home (Ephesians 5:22). As a child, I was under the authority of my parents and teachers, but if I did not learn to respect that, I would be struggling now as an adult to respect authority at work and in marriage. As children of God, He also places us in a church family where we respect the authority of leaders there, according to God's Word. We honour people not because they are perfect, but because we honour the God who allowed them to hold those positions. He is all-knowing and has a plan bigger than what we can see. The Bible even tells us to respect the king and government authorities, because "there is no authority except from God, and the authorities that exist are appointed by God" (Romans 13). They are also answerable to God for the decisions they make and how they look after the people they lead.

We can lead from the back by being good examples to those around us. The God who sees all things will surely reward even the smallest good deeds done in secret and promote us at the right time. I love the story of Joseph, recorded in the book of Genesis in the Bible. He started as a slave in Egypt, but the Spirit of excellence in him led him to be the head of Portiphar's household servants and a leader even when he ended up in prison for resisting the temptation to sleep with Portiphar's wife. He eventually became ruler of Egypt, second only to Pharoah, at a time when he had matured enough to forgive those who sold him into slavery. I am always encouraged by the fact that, even though it took years for God's promise of greatness for Joseph to happen, he lived many more years after that enjoying the success. Many lives were saved from famine because of him.

It is never too late to go for our dreams. It does take boldness and humility, courage and wisdom, but nothing is impossible for those who believe. Being in a place of power and responsibility is not to be taken for granted, and should not be abused. We should be truly grateful whenever we are given a chance to lead and influence others, whether in a small group or global setting. It is not always because we are the most qualified but by God's grace and mercy. People often ask "Why me?!" when something bad happens, but I have yet to see people who ask this when they experience undeserved favour. Somehow humans feel entitled to a problem-free life. We should never take for granted the blessings and opportunities we get, because not everyone gets them. The impact we have as leaders can have long-lasting effects, whether positive or negative, so leadership is a huge responsibility that we must think carefully about before accepting. Leaders must keep growing and improving themselves, so they do not mislead others. The fact that people are supporting and following a leader should not become a source of pride, but of responsibility, because we need to treat others as we want to be treated. Remember that feeling happy and safe is an important human desire, and it is a blessing to be in positions of power that can help make that happen for others.

Being good at something

I remember feeling frustrated as a GP trainee whenever people asked why I "did not want to specialise". It was often because people did not realise that General Practice (Family Medicine) is a speciality in itself. People prefer to see junior doctors training to become cardiologists (heart specialists) or brain surgeons but struggle to understand why someone like me would want to be a "generalist", especially after all the huge hurdles we have to overcome as immigrant professionals. In fact, I have heard of people speaking rudely to GPs, wanting to be referred to the "proper consultant" in hospital. Thankfully, I am confident and happy with my career choice, which has allowed me to do what is best for my personality and skills. General Practice requires me to have a broad base of medical knowledge, which allows me to help more people and feel relevant in the community.

I remember admiring how my husband, who is a community pharmacist, can advise friends and family about simple ailments and common conditions, while I had no idea what to do about a simple annoying rash, even though I was working in a surgical speciality helping people with cancer. Working in General Practice allows me to see and treat the common problems people have, while being aware of signs of the rare and serious conditions, which need to be referred on. We do a lot of chronic disease management, screening/prevention programmes, as well as treatment of infections and diseases that could otherwise be fatal if everyone had to wait for hospital appointments. I love working in the UK National Health Service (NHS) where healthcare is free at the point of delivery. Despite the problems and limited resources, we still provide better care than is available in many countries around the world, and I believe this is thanks to the thousands of GPs who have broad knowledge to provide "cradle to grave" care, and the wider multidisciplinary teams we work with.

Many GPs develop special interests over the course of their careers, and I have naturally tended towards mental health because of my unusually long psychiatry experience during my training years. I also intentionally built on that experience by shadowing psychiatry clinics after I became a qualified GP, and later took on a rewarding county-wide mental health "GP in Psychiatry" role. I have also been the mental health lead in practices where I work, which often leads to more exposure to mental health cases. It was a case of practising what I preach when I decided to build my special interest around things I am naturally good at, which fit in with my life's purpose. I know people struggle with the idea of finding your purpose, but I don't think it is as complicated as we make it sound. The clues are usually in our personality, interests and strengths.

Someone once said that the thing that annoys you the most is the problem you were created to solve. I know that it breaks my heart to see people making poor choices due to ignorance, giving up in the face of challenges and struggling mentally, so I am grateful to be able to help in that way through my medical work and writing. It also makes sense to build on subjects we are naturally good at, rather than trying to be experts in subjects we find very challenging - which is why mathematics-related jobs were never an option for me! We can achieve anything when we put our minds to it, but we do not want to be constantly on an uphill struggle for the rest of our lives. I put in the effort to do well in maths at school, but it would have been unwise to go on to become a statistician, for example. When people are praised for things they excel at, no one really cares if they started from level zero to become experts or if they just built up their natural talent to become respected experts. We can build on our natural interests and strengths to shine bright and bring solutions, instead of trying to be someone else. Watching the achievements of people like Serena Williams and Usain Bolt reminds me of how much we can achieve with talent and hard work put together.

Adding value

We become good at what we do, not just to feel good in ourselves, but to contribute positively to the world around us. It takes time, effort and a lot of learning to become very good at something. People are not born experts, and hard work will eventually trump talent if the talented person does not keep improving themself and putting in the work needed. We can see that already with the social media craze for having more and more followers, when people who are excellent at what they do might appear to have fewer followers than someone who spends all their time "creating content" for their social media page to gain more attention. We then have to recognise that the effort being rewarded there is the content creation effort rather than the actual level of expertise. It is also a case of choosing where we feel more drawn to add value - in the real world or online. I have seen people who are busy doing great work offline (while having little or no online presence) and others who fill up all social media platforms with the little they have achieved. Social media has its benefits, but I have come to realise that it is worth delegating the publicity aspect to people who are good at that so that we can spend time doing what we love, while maintaining a good online presence as well - if that is important or relevant for what we do.

We add value when we make a positive impact on those who come in contact with us or our services. We add value when we solve problems and share ideas. I remember hearing a sobering quote about how people will remember us for the problems we solved *and* created. While trying to add value and solve problems, we need to be sure that we are not also creating worse problems. Doctors have to balance this often when we prescribe helpful medications with consideration for possible side effects. Some problems might be difficult to foresee until new ideas are implemented, but if it is within our power, we can try to also solve the problems we create in the process of adding value so that we do not leave our mess for someone else to fix. We are all enjoying the fast devices and communication the internet provides, but there have also been problems related to such technological advances, especially in young people today, who struggle to have proper conversations and relationships. I think that there is very little we can do to shield our little ones from social media and the internet, but we can educate them on the risks, and support them to make good choices.

As a mother, I think that adding value to my family is not about doing everything for my children but empowering them to be more independent and confident as they grow up. We all want to feel significant and valued - even children do. That adds to our sense of power and control. We can add value easily here by choosing our words wisely at home and also in the workplace, so that people feel encouraged or motivated, rather than deflated, after spending time with us. Work is not just about the money. We see people leave well-paying jobs to chase more satisfying hobbies and interests because they want to feel significant and relevant in the big wide world. Even though we all want to feel valued, people sometimes have limited choices when it comes to their work and career because of other choices they have made, such as education/training, family and financial commitments - I share more about this in my book, *Money and Mental Wellbeing*. It is a beautiful thing when we can find satisfaction and add value to others through the activities of our everyday lives. I feel so blessed to have found a form of this balance now and to be helping others to do the same.

Unsung Heroes

Success is measured differently by different people, which is why it is good to have our own ideas of what success looks like for us. We cannot depend on worldly commendation to determine if we have been successful because people can be fickle and change their minds easily. There was a time when having mansions, designer clothes and brand-new cars were the measure of success, but it is now common to see wealthy people proudly living minimalist lifestyles. Doctors used to be praised for working almost 100 hours a week and appearing to manage well without sleep, but living like that is now seen as having a poor quality of life with a higher risk of heart disease and burnout. There was a time when a woman's worth was measured by the number of children she had and how well she hosted others for meals in her matrimonial home, but there are now many happy wives who do not know how to cook and choose not to have children. Trying too hard to fit into societal norms can sometimes lead to comparison and depression that will not have been worth it when we look back years later.

I look back now to my days in medical school when it was unpopular to want to become a GP. Only two of us put our hands up to show interest in this speciality when a lecturer asked a class of over 100 medical students what we wanted to specialise in. Most people wanted to do the glamorous medical and surgical specialities in hospitals, and I remember wanting to become a surgeon myself at the start of medical school. I am so grateful now for the tough season of my life in 2007 when I had to take a year out of medical school due to financial difficulties and travel back to Nigeria in tears. That season made me discover more about myself and the kind of life I wanted. It was at that time that I wrote my first book, *Fortitude*, and founded *Forte Charity for Inspiration*. I realised that I enjoy working in the community, and would prefer the kind of career and lifestyle that General Practice offers. Around half of medical students end up in General Practice. Many of my medical colleagues ended up changing their minds, some even halfway through other speciality training, and after struggling with exams and jobs in specialities that did not suit their personalities or life circumstances. I am incredibly proud of and grateful for medical colleagues who enjoy and succeed in hospital specialities because they make the healthcare team complete. Although it was a tough time in my life when I struggled financially in medical school, the resilience and wisdom I gained in that season have stood me in good stead for life as a doctor. Indeed, "all things work together for good for those who love God" (Romans 8:28). Having this perspective helps us to be less stressed in the face of challenges.

People like to think that they know what success looks like, but we should not be deceived into judging success superficially. Many people are doing great jobs in different sectors with little recognition for their contribution until they are no longer there. I heard of a mental health charity volunteer who had to re-open a service because there were sadly two suicides and the imprisonment of one of their clients for murder committed when the service closed down. Just by being there to listen and support people with mental health problems, the volunteer was having such a powerful impact on the community, preventing distress, crime and suicide. There are also so many people caring for relatives at home, preventing deaths and hospital admissions that we will never hear about. I have so much respect also for parents looking after children with special needs and learning disabilities, knowing that their child might never gain full independence and leave home like others. I also think of the underpaid junior staff in so many companies that keep our economy going, as well as the stay-at-home parents who support their spouses to have great careers. They may never get loud praise and recognition but should be just as proud of how powerful their contributions are.

Roll with the changes

Although we talk about seasons of life and career where there is hardly any recognition for what we do, I believe that if we keep doing our best and growing in our roles, we will eventually get the praise we deserve. It is often said that the only constant in life is change. If we are to remain relevant in today's world, we have to be able to deal with change positively. Change can be uncomfortable and sometimes painful, but if we see the opportunities rather than the hindrances, we can reap benefits from even the most unexpected changes. I often have to reassess my ways of working when there have been changes in my family life in order to stay productive, even in the tough seasons. There have been seasons when it was better to do my medical work in the mornings, to allow time for school runs in the afternoon and family time in the evenings. Now my children are older, I can afford to do a few longer days and still have time with my family as the children are no longer asleep by 7 pm. There were, of course, financial implications for working part-time, but I am happy with the choices I made for that stage of life because I like to balance my priorities and be there for the family I choose to have.

There might be seasons in life where we have to work more hours, stretch ourselves or pay more bills, which can be hard - for example, for someone who never had to work because their spouse was earning enough for the family, or someone who has to retrain for a new career after redundancy. Instead of complaining and giving up, we can roll with the punches and rise to the challenge. As I have found over time, those challenges are opportunities for growth and praise when we manoeuvre the obstacles successfully. People like to celebrate success, but there will be nothing to celebrate and we cannot be overcomers if there is nothing to overcome. The phrase "roll with the punches" comes from boxing, because we are like boxers moving tactfully to lessen the impact of life's punches when we adapt well to difficult situations and setbacks. Adapting does not mean changing our whole lives because something has "gone wrong in our plan". We can stay focused on our goals and true to our vision while adapting to changing circumstances. I remember having to study Anatomy as a first degree when I did not get into medical school at 18. I could have easily carried on to develop my career as a scientist, especially because I was invited for an interview for a job in Cambridge after that degree. It was a hard decision, considering my financial situation, but I did all I could to stay focused on my goal of becoming a medical doctor, even if it meant working as a carer to pay my rent and having no money for trips abroad while my friends were travelling.

Some changes are temporary and we can hang in there for the storm to pass, but some changes are more permanent, for example, the loss of a loved one or a chronic illness diagnosis. It is hard to find the strength to deal with such issues especially when it brings sudden change and questions our identity. I often find strength in knowing that none of it is a surprise to God and He will see me through. Also, because my true identity is in Christ, and He never changes, I can maintain the peace within and navigate the new scenario with God's help. On a practical note, I would take some time to process the change and what it means for my life going forward, accept what I cannot change and resist what is unacceptable to me as a child of God so that I can continue enjoying the abundant life God has for me. I remember praying about my husband's health when we first got married because he was having terrible sickle cell crises almost every six months when I met him. Even though I understand the cause and prognosis for this, as a medical doctor, I chose not to accept a life of recurrent hospital admissions for my husband. The Holy Bible tells me that there is healing power in Christ and I have seen it for myself in our lives. When health challenges came up, which have been rare in the past 14 years (thank God!), we reschedule what needs to be rescheduled in our calendars, inform whoever needs to be informed of his admission and trust God for strength and healing, as we roll with the punches. Having faith does not mean refusing medication and medical help, but knowing that healing comes from God. We do not give up on our faith or stop praising our Maker, we do not extrapolate to say that life is all bad, and we certainly do not sit around feeling sorry for ourselves, because we know that we still have so much to be grateful for, no matter what. We know that sickle cell disease can be debilitating and we have seen people with terrible complications of the condition, so I am proud of my husband for looking beyond himself to set up a platform called *Sickle Cell Mentorship* to support others to live well with the condition.

Sometimes the best way to handle change is to think beyond ourselves to help those who might be suffering worse than we are. The things we take for granted might be just what some-one else is praying for. My husband is a practising community pharmacist and has stories of children with Sickle Cell Disease who see him and are excited to meet a professional who knows what it feels like to suffer severely painful sickle cell crises, miss school and still have to pass important exams. Remembering that our successful handling of challenges and change is not just for ourselves but for many others looking up to us helps us to find the strength to keep going. As a GP partner, I often have to watch the language I use when talking about changes to NHS policy and requirements from us as a GP surgery, so as not to drain energy from our staff who may also be strug-gling with the implementation of (sometimes sudden) changes, such as the need to administer thousands of vaccines to our patients within a few weeks in flu season, increase in de-mand for appointments and harder targets, funding cuts and staff shortages. It is better to be realistic, proactive and hope-ful about change so that we come out stronger.

CHAPTER 2
The Power of Today

Be here now

How many times do we catch ourselves wishing our lives away, wanting what comes next and not enjoying the moments? When I was in school, I could not wait to start working. Now I am working, I long for time to study or write. The things we once prayed for are now reality, yet we forget how badly we used to want them. I often remind myself of this when I find myself getting irritated at little children messing up my tidy house. When I got married at age 26, I was in the third year of medical school, so we decided not to have children until I completed the four-year graduate-entry medical course. It was quite a change going from a shared student house to a three-bedroom terraced house with my husband. Thankfully, he is not an untidy man, so we enjoyed having our own space.

I remember our first house had such a tiny kitchen, that two people could not be in it without brushing past each other.

Our friends used to joke that it was great for getting newlyweds to make up after a fight. Even though it was a small, old, rented house, we decorated it the best we could and hosted several guests for meals there, as we still enjoy doing. We decided to enjoy what we had and not let the limitations of that house stop us from living the life we wanted. We love hosting, so we did not let the size of that house stop us from joining the open home rota at church, which involved hosting the whole (small) church for lunch after Sunday morning meetings - it was our turn about one in ten Sundays. The church was very considerate and there would usually be fewer people in attendance if they knew that it was at a smaller house. In the summer, we managed to host more people because my husband took good care of the garden, making it a lovely social space when the weather was good. We still talk about how people who treat a small rented house well will do the same if they get to buy a big house, but people who treat a rented or small house badly will not suddenly become tidy and house-proud even if they are given a big mansion. Jesus talked about how someone who is faithful with a little will be faithful with much, but for those who do not look after the "little" they have, even that will be taken away from them. Being present is not just about enjoying the fun moments of life, but being aware of the blessings, opportunities and resources we have now, so we can use them well, not just waiting till we get something better.

When I finished medical school in 2012, I decided that I wanted to work for one year first to ensure that I had full registration with the UK General Medical Council (GMC) before getting pregnant. We were enjoying our marriage and my dear husband was not bothered about whether we had children or not. He had been so traumatised after watching a childbirth (with episiotomy) video when he came to one of my medical school lectures, that he told me that we did not have to have children! I had told God (and everyone who cared to know) right from my childhood in Nigeria, that I wanted to have two children - a daughter, then a son, two years apart. I think it came from watching my parents and aunties who mostly had four children, and deciding that I did not want such a full house when raising my children. I figured I could always adopt more later if I wanted, and there were already many needy children in the world. I know many people have changed their minds about how many children they want over the years, but somehow I have remained firm on this despite the gorgeous babies I see at work that sometimes tempt me to consider having another one. As long as people are happy and can cope with the responsibility, I think they can have whatever number of children they want.

My school friends used to say that I would never find a Nigerian man who would want only two children, because it was popular to have four children in Nigeria in the 80s, but life has changed a lot since then. I met my husband in England and it is now very common for couples to have two children. This is why I have learned to do what works for me and my relationship with God, not what everyone else is doing. I have always known that my Maker has a great plan for my life, which I am still discovering. God very kindly gave me the two lovely children I wanted - almost exactly two years apart, but there was a period when I was trying to get pregnant after my Foundation Year one as a junior doctor and it was not happening, You can imagine how hard that must have been for someone who likes to plan ahead and feel in control. We prayed and did everything right medically but I was still not pregnant six months later. All sorts of thoughts start to run through your mind as a woman of 29 struggling to conceive. I remembered how my mum had me at age 22 and how fertility declines with age. I wondered if it might end up becoming a journey of 21 years as it was for my uncle or a case of getting pregnant at 90 like Sarah in the Bible. I believed I would have children one day - God does not always tell us *when* exactly He will do something, but we can trust that it *will* happen if He said it.

I had to choose to enjoy my life while waiting so that I did not end up ruining the beautiful marriage and friendships I already had. Other friends and relatives were having babies within a year of getting married, and I had to try to be happy for them, intentionally enjoying the moments of waiting for mine. I wondered if the research was wrong and if the long-acting reversible contraception I used had affected me badly. I often say that statistics mean nothing for the one. Considering I only started using contraception when we got married three years prior, I found comfort in knowing from my medical work that other women used contraception from age 15 and still had babies at 30. They do say that comparison is the thief of joy. I had to be careful not to start comparing myself to anyone and just keep trusting God while we waited. Working in the local hospital as a junior doctor (doing long on-call shifts) was getting stressful, and I sometimes got angry that I was not yet on maternity leave.

Words are powerful - I had to choose to keep speaking positively, so I would not get anxious or depressed. I even bought some cute baby clothes on sale because I focused on faith, not fear. I continued to do my medical and charity work well, being present in what we had, not just longing for what was not yet here. Some days were very difficult and I am not sure how well I would have coped if the waiting lasted much longer, but I was so happy to finally have conceived after 11 months of trying. God never gives us more than we can bear. We know that 90% of healthy couples will conceive with regular unprotected sexual intercourse within two years of trying, but the problem is that you do not know at the start if you are one of the majority that will, or whether you might end up needing medical assistance, which is a totally different, challenging emotional journey. To be able to enjoy the present, without losing our peace and power, we have to choose to believe not fear; to trust that even in the worst-case scenario, God will work it all out for good. Losing our peace makes us lose the power to be productive in the period of waiting - which could be 11 months or 11 years. I would hate to have looked back on that time after getting pregnant and wondered why I wasted it doing nothing else. Having a higher perspective helps us to see that, in the grand scheme of things, waiting is not that bad because there is a correct time and season for everything. God is a good Father and gives us what we need at the perfect time, just like a sensible father would only give his son a car to drive when it is safe to do so not when he is eleven years old. The conception delay meant that I qualified for maternity pay when I took time off to have the baby, I was mature enough to cope with parenting and my daughter will probably do things that only people born in 2014 were meant to do! Now when I get irritated by children being naughty, I remind myself how much I prayed to have them and praise God for the privilege of raising them.

Self-control

I think the idea of having self-control is one of the main reasons why I do not drink alcohol. Apart from the fact that my body reacts badly to it, I personally do not like the thought of being controlled by anything other than the leading of God's Holy Spirit. Jesus miraculously turned water into wine, so we know that drinking alcohol is not wrong, but excessive alcohol use is not healthy or wise. When we were younger, it was funny to hear about people getting drunk on a night out and doing things they are not proud of. It is surprising that some people still do this even in their 40s and older. I do not think that it is wrong to go out and have fun, but too much of anything is not good. The damage that excess alcohol does to the brain, nerves and liver is not worth the "fun". Some people drink to forget their sorrows, but it is better to face our problems because they will still be there (and probably be worse) after the drunkenness clears. Some people do not drink to get drunk but regularly exceed the safe weekly alcohol limit, slowly damaging their organs and shortening their lifespan. Knowing that alcohol is a depressant is another reason to avoid having alcohol as part of our routine if we want to look after our mental health. It is sad to see how popular the idea of having "a large glass of wine after putting children to bed" has become among young mums in the Western world. Alcoholism is not just a problem of the poor and deprived, but of the wealthy who can afford even stronger varieties and pretend that they are not addicted. It does not take much to find oneself regularly drinking over the recommended safe weekly limit for alcohol. The Bible warns us to not be drunk with wine (Ephesians 5:18) but to be full of the Holy Spirit, because the fruit of the Spirit is love, joy, peace, patience, kindness, goodness, faithfulness, gentleness and self-control (Galatians 5:22) - and who would not want these?

If we cannot control ourselves, how can we hope to manage anyone else well? People are impressed by managerial positions, leadership and titles, but a manager who cannot control himself - his temper, his speech, his habits, his thoughts and his reactions will soon end up in ruin. In James 3, the Bible says that "if we could control our tongues, we would be perfect and could also control ourselves in every other way" but the writer acknowledges how hard this is, and that is why we need God's help every day. We all make mistakes and have to keep renewing our minds if we are to make progress in this area. For anyone who thinks they have achieved wisdom and understand God's ways, James advises to "prove it by living an honourable life, doing good works with the humility that comes from wisdom" and we know that God is willing to give wisdom to anyone who asks (James 1:5). We can learn wisdom by listening to wise people and filling our minds with the right things. The mouth speaks from what the heart contains. If we want to have self-control in the area of speech, it will be wise to surround ourselves with people who speak well, not gossips, grumblers, liars and those who constantly use foul language. We never know who is listening. People have incriminated themselves, caused wars and even saved nations by the words of their mouths. There is real power in learning to think before we speak.

Some people blame their surroundings, upbringing and friends for their lack of self-control, but it is up to us to change our friends and surroundings if they are not fit for purpose. We can choose to get help to learn and unlearn ways of thinking and doing things. People might even choose to move to a completely different city to change their lives if they have grown up around negativity and habits that they struggle to break. Patients sometimes tell me about how hard it is to resist going back to a life of drugs or other unhealthy habits, especially on stressful days, after enjoying the benefits of freedom for months. The broad answer is to avoid the temptation and trigger stations in the first place, and change the way we think - which is what we try to achieve through Cognitive Behavioural Therapy (CBT). Jesus said that if your eye causes you to sin, pluck it out! That is a metaphor for removing anything (no matter how painful the separation) that deters you from living the eternal life God created you to live. We are what we think, so instead of regularly watching violence, for example, and wondering why one has no self-control when angry, it is better to choose wisely what we see and hear, so that only good comes out of us. As long as I surround myself with unhealthy snacks and people who have unhealthy eating habits, weight loss will continue to be a struggle. We set boundaries for ourselves and avoid certain things, not always because they are bad in themselves, but because it is wise to intentionally avoid the trouble, sickness or stress those things might lead to.

Power over time

It is interesting how we often talk about time flying by like it is something we are surprised about. The principle has been the same since before we were born - day follows night. The Bible says in the book of Ecclesiastes that there is “a time for everything”. Apart from the amazing miracle recorded in the

Bible where God kept the sun up for a full day for Joshua to win a battle after he prayed, we know that the daylight hours and calendar months are standard for wherever we live. What we do with them is what makes the difference. Whatever time we spend on one thing is time not available for something else. Time is a precious and limited resource, which is frankly more important than money. When we learn to manage our time well, there is no limit to how far we can go. Whether we get to live 100 years or 50 years, it is what we did with the time that matters, not the length of it. Even a child begins to show evidence of self-will from only a few months old. A baby can decide to keep you seated for over one hour feeding her if she refuses to open her mouth, or she can comply and let you finish in five minutes. We too, as adults, can decide what to permit and what not to permit with our time.

It is a shame when we leave the management of our time to chance and look back to see how much was actually wasted. I wake up each day with an idea of all the things I would like to achieve that day, which is usually confirmed after spending some time with God through prayer. I commit my day to God and trust Him to make it fruitful. I can surely testify that I cannot remember when last I had a "bad day" because God does not fail. Even when something bad happens, I usually see God turn it around for my good. I remember times when I have been so worried driving in bad traffic and wondering why God let that happen, only to get somewhere and find out that I arrived at just the perfect time for something good, because of the delay. I cannot even imagine the number of accidents and disasters God protected me from when He allowed delays and incidents that I might have felt were a waste of time. There have also been times when I felt led by

God's Holy Spirit to leave a task till later, only to find that new information comes in before I sit down to face it, and that new information means that I do not need to do that task anymore or the solution is much clearer. God knows all I have in my diary as well as everything else going on elsewhere that I do not know - He always provides the right help and connections. Taking time to speak to someone or do something He wants me to do has never been a regret, even on a busy day, because He makes up for it in other ways. Sometimes a meeting I was rushing for gets cancelled and I can rest sooner than planned.

Being intentional with our time, while trusting the Owner of time and eternity is a great way to have power over time. We are the ones who end up living with the consequences of the choices we make, so we should not be eager to delegate the responsibility of the management of our time to anyone else. We always have a choice, even when it comes to work. Any manager who sees a proactive worker using their time well will be keen to let that worker manage their time more independently because the results will speak for themselves. We should be aware of the impact on our time when we agree to take on any job or responsibility. The time you spend doing that will mean less time to spend with your family or pursuing other interests unless you have managed to merge them into your work. We need to balance the need to get paid with the need for sleep, growth and relaxation. I sometimes hear people complaining that their 9-5 job stops them from doing what they really want to do with their time, but I remind them that there are 16 hours left after work, so you can do it if you really want to. We sometimes forget to calculate the time spent on phones, social media, sitting around idly, talking to people, cleaning, watching TV and lying in bed. All of it counts towards our 24 hours and our lives are a result of how we have been using our time. Time flies, but you are the pilot.

Time management patterns that worked years ago may not be useful now. If you used to stay in bed for 10 hours as a student and still managed to succeed as a first-class student, you cannot keep doing that now that you also have a job and family, and expect to have the same level of success in life. We need to keep re-inventing ourselves and doing what works for new seasons of life. I am always impressed by entertainers and professionals who manage to stay relevant across generations because of how they rebrand themselves and keep going with the new demands of the industry. When we refuse to reflect and review our time management regularly, we can end up stale and lose the will to live. I was sad to hear about a 100-year-old woman who used to be upset about waking up because she could not wait to die. Understandably, she was sad that most of her friends and family had died, but I believe that as long as we have breath and good cognition, we can still enjoy life by being a blessing to others. I can imagine how many people would have loved to hear her stories from long ago or to see her handiwork if she tried to keep herself occupied somehow. Sadly, some people much younger than that are also feeling just as aimless in life because every day is the same, achieving almost nothing. We can choose to take control of our time and make each day a productive one when we see things from a better viewpoint of a world that needs the gifts in us.

Happiness over stress

When I became busier as a GP partner, I started a podcast because there was no time for writing regular articles like I used to. I scheduled my time to allow for monthly recording of groups of my weekly podcasts, as an outlet which was great for my mental health and vision. I called it "Afiniki's Happiness Over Stress Podcast", from the subtitle of my book, *Life Without Coffee*. The phrase reminds me that it is our choice whether to be happy or stressed, whatever situation we find ourselves in, and the choice gives us power through managing our attitude and reaction to the curve balls that life throws at us. A famous Christian speaker used to say that we can be powerful or pitiful, but we cannot be both. This was something that God showed her at a time when she was dwelling on the traumatic experiences of her past, being difficult to live with and struggling to love others well. Today is a gift that we cannot recover when it is gone. We can choose to enjoy what is working now or dwell on things we cannot change, which can lead to frustration and bitterness. No matter how difficult life is, there will always be something positive we can focus on to kindle some gratitude in our hearts, even if it is just the fact that we are still alive. We can then find peace in knowing that the giver of the blessing we are not taking for granted (life) can do much more when we persevere in faith. I would rather believe this and have positive energy to get through my days than let myself feel so hopeless and pitiful that I have no energy to do what is possible today, which might be the key to getting out of the tough situation. Sometimes we have to do what is good for our mental health when we do not feel like it so that our mental health and motivation will improve.

People sometimes argue that they cannot help how they feel, but living from a higher perspective helps us to know that we are the bosses of our minds. When we notice negative and unhelpful thoughts creep in, we quickly get rid of them by focusing on positive things. Some people use affirmations, scriptures, motivational quotes and music to tell their minds what to think. It sometimes even involves physically going somewhere to hear what we *need* to hear, not what we want to hear. Leaving our minds blank will often turn an idle mind into the devil's workshop. I focus my mind on the truth of God's word rather than the lies and worries the world throws at us. There is often positive Christian music playing in my car and house as I go about my business. One of my favourite verses, which I say daily, is "For God has not given us a spirit of fear, but of power, of love and a sound mind" (2 Timothy 1:7). Most of the things people worry about do not eventually happen, and those that happen are probably not as bad as we imagined. There is so much power in the mind and when we realise that faith works, we can choose to believe for good things and not negative things. When we keep saying and expecting negative outcomes, due to fear and worry, it is no surprise that we get a life full of such. Whether people are Christians or not, I have noticed that words are indeed powerful, and people who speak and expect positive things are usually more successful.

Happiness over stress is not just about positive thinking, but doing the things that help us to maintain that power in our minds, from which we get the energy to be productive in all areas of life. When we are stressed, everything feels like a chore. The time we should be enjoying with our family and friends turns into arguments and moaning sessions, we then suffer poor sleep and become even grumpier at work, leading to more workplace conflict and sometimes financial repercussions due to lack of work or promotions. We all get stressful days when it is a real struggle to stay positive, and it is easy to stay down when things go wrong. Choosing happiness over stress is about taking back power over those circumstances (to not allow them to get us depressed or anxious) by looking at the bigger picture of life and eternity to stay hopeful. I sometimes remind myself that something is just a ten-minute problem or a one-year problem, so I do not let it ruin my whole day. Giving the problem an estimated time frame helps us to see how small it really is compared to the rest of our lives. I have had jobs that involved working with very unpleasant people. Instead of letting them ruin my life and personality, I remind myself that I am only there for six months and do what I can each day to get through, thanking God that time does fly by. I like the saying, "If you do not like where you are - move! You are not a tree". Mine were fixed medical rotations that I had to do for my GP training, but I could have applied for other jobs elsewhere if they weren't. I could have also chosen to drop out of GP training - I am glad I did not. Most people can find a better job or house within a year or two, if they improve themselves and set their minds to it. I have often looked back on those seasons and realised that I learned a lot, especially when God did not allow me to get out of the situation as quickly as I wanted to. The thing I thought was trying to break me, had made me a stronger person. We can humble ourselves to learn life lessons from tough times fast so we can move on to greater things. God is not more concerned about our comfort than our growth, so life will always have challenges. I did not smile all day on the tough days, but I did not let the situation take away my peace and power.

Love is the greatest

The Bible tells us that "God is love" (1 John 4:8), so when I hear some descriptions of love referring to lust, sex, attraction, greed or selfishness, it makes me sad that we do not truly understand the power of love. Love is more powerful than money, position, passion and fame. This is why people often feel empty even after acquiring all the wealth they thought would make them happy. There is nothing wrong with being wealthy but it is sad when money is the most important thing in one's life. Yes, money can be a tool to make things happen but that should not become our identity or idol if we want to navigate life from a higher perspective. We should own money and not let money own us. A good way to understand this is to imagine the hole there would be in your heart if you lost all your money or job, versus if your relationship with someone ended. Do we value people more than things? Even if we are tempted to, we can choose to prioritise souls more than riches, as the all-knowing God does. When we do things our way and pursue temporal physical things, we might learn the hard way that the most valuable things in life are unseen and eternal.

I find it such a blessing that Jesus simplified it for us - love God and love people. Actually, He said, "*Love the Lord your God with all your soul and with all your mind and with all your strength. The second is this, love your neighbour as yourself. There is no commandment greater than these.*" (Mark 12: 30-31) People are changed positively by the power of love. Being judgemental, scary or bossy only damages them. We have seen many times throughout history how good overcomes evil because God is love and God is good, so there is no greater power. Loving people is not the same as doing good works, giving to charity or being polite, which can all be evidence of love. When we love people we genuinely care for their well-being and want the best for them, even if they do not appreciate us for it. It is possible to do the motions without really caring for people, but the Apostle Paul said that all our good works count for nothing if we do not have love. Love is the motive that makes it all worthwhile. Jesus showed us sacrificial love when He left His glorious place in heaven to live with and die for mere mortals so that we can have the chance to live forever with Him when we put our faith in the risen Christ. This explains the eternity-seeking, God-shaped hole in our hearts, that longs for more, even after people gain all the money and power they want.

Some people figure this out sooner in life, while others only discover this on their deathbeds with regret. We want to be powerful, not pitiful, but I believe the greatest power is not in work titles, marriage, money, politics, royalty, fame, talent, skill, physical strength or academic qualifications. There is real power in accepting and showing God's love which is free to all, to give us a great life on this earth and for eternity. I am still learning to walk in God's love as I go about different aspects of my life, as I would not want it all to be worth nothing in the end because I did not do things out of love. It can be easy to have a condescending or judgemental attitude when in a position to help others, but I pray to always have compassion and grace in my heart, knowing that we are all made different and have different paths in life. I am yet to see where love was not the best solution. We can make better decisions when we love ourselves and love others with wisdom and humility. Loving my parents as a child would make me honour and obey them to stay out of trouble, loving myself as a teenager would keep me away from dangerous drugs, relationships and habits, loving myself as an adult would help me make better spending, relationship and work decisions, loving my friends would help me to speak the truth as needed and make time for them, loving my neighbours would make me check on them and share what I have, loving my country helps me to be law-abiding and considerate of others, loving my husband helps me to forgive and see the best in him, loving my staff helps me to focus less on money and more on their wellbeing and a peaceful workplace, loving my patients would help me to overlook their frustration/manner and show compassion, loving my managers would help me see them as people not just actions and imperfections, loving my children motivates me to be a good role model for them, and loving God gives me the strength to serve Him every day, even when it seems foolish or unpopular. Living a life of love does not mean that I am perfect, but I will keep doing my best to grow in love.

Faith that moves mountains

The Bible talks about having child-like faith and defines faith as the "assurance of things hoped for and the evidence of things not seen" (Hebrews 11:1). We all believe in something, whether we want to admit it or not. I choose to believe in one greater than myself because I know that I cannot win in this life without God. Some people lose faith in God because they expect Him to be like a genie granting our every wish and giving us trouble-free lives. The interesting thing is that Jesus never promised that. He told us clearly that there will be troubles in this life, but He has overcome, making us "more than conquerors" in Him. The Bible tells us that temptation and evil do not come from God but as a consequence of the fallen state of our sinful world. When we put our faith in Jesus, we get to live a victorious life, despite the evil around us. We start to see also that "all things are possible for him who believes", as the Bible says.

1 John 5:14-15 says, "*This is the confidence we have in approaching God: that if we ask anything according to His will, He hears us. And if we know that He hears us—whatever we ask—we know that we have what we asked of Him*". As people who have surrendered our lives to God, what we want more than our desires is for God's will to be done, so when we pray and feel like things have not gone how we wanted or in our time frame, we can trust that God's will is better and greater than ours. As children of God, we do not exalt our desire for anything higher than our desire to please God - that is idolatry, which we are advised against in 1 John 5: 20-21, "*And we know that the Son of God has come and has given us understanding, so that we may know Him who is true; and we are in Him who is true, in His Son Jesus Christ. He is the true God and eternal life. Little children, keep yourselves from idols.*" The Bible shows us that God is more interested in the humility and faith in our hearts than in repetitive prayers and religious rituals, even though those actions might help build our faith and discipline. Jesus said that if we have faith as small as a mustard seed, we can move mountains. Now, that is power! Mountains refer to the impossible situations we come across in life, many of which I have seen God change through faith. Although in His infinite wisdom, He might empower us to climb over the mountain rather than move it.

I remember how my dream of becoming a British medical doctor as a girl from a minority tribe in Nigeria was a matter of faith. Marrying a man with sickle cell disease because I believe God said to do so, even though medical and common sense goes against it, is surely a matter of faith in God. As a child in Nigeria, I learned to trust God that there would not be a power cut when I needed to study or iron my school uniform, that my parents would be able to pay my fees in time for end-of-term exams, that we would travel safely on some dangerous roads, and for many other things that helped to strengthen my faith. As an adult now, I try not to take the simple things of life for granted just because I now live in England with safe roads, constant electricity and no school fees to pay for my school-age children. I remember to exercise my child-like faith when faced with challenges that make others give up. God gave us miraculous provision for the mortgage deposit for our first house, supernatural health and strength even with a diagnosis of sickle cell disease, problem-free pregnancies and childbirths in spite of my family history, provision of work and friends wherever we go, and so many more blessings I cannot list here. I have seen irreparable marriages restored, wayward children repent and businesses prosper because someone chose to have faith and pray. I wrote about the ups and downs of my faith when trying to move house in my book, *2020 Year of Plenty*, and was disappointed to have to end the book with no big story of how God eventually brought the perfect buyer for our first house. I believe God wanted me to learn that the ending we know is usually not the real ending of a story where God is involved. The story of my book finished in December 2020 but by May 2021 God provided us with a new house, in addition to the one we wanted to sell. I would never have thought that we would have been financially able to move without selling the first house, but God works in His own timing and does what is best for us. His plan is always better if only we will wait. Our property story has not ended and I am excited about living a life of faith, where nothing is impossible.

One preacher described our relationship with God as a woman dating a wealthy man. While dating him, she can see all his properties but has no rights to them until she fully commits to him in marriage. I have realised that knowing about God is very different from fully living for Him. We get the full benefits of peace, joy and victorious living in Christ when we totally surrender our lives to God and trust His plan for us. It is part of my choosing happiness over stress to go with the winning team - Jesus never fails. There is power in prayer, but we cannot be double-minded or "on the fence" with God if we want a fulfilled spiritual life. The Bible says that a double-minded person should not expect to receive anything from God (James 1). God graciously shines His sun on the good and evil, but there are greater blessings that only sons and daughters can enjoy. There are many other spiritual powers in this world, but I choose to believe in the one true God, and His Son Jesus Christ, whose power works mightily in and through me for good. The proof of the power is in what it can accomplish. I have seen many miracles and lives turned around for good by the power of God, so I cannot write a book about power without talking about the most powerful One. Respect for and faith in a great God has definitely allowed me to have peace, joy and hope in my life.

Never the same

Someone once said that it is only a fool who thinks that things will always remain as they are. This quote reminds me that life is always changing, so even in the good times, I must not forget to plan - just like the Egyptians saved in their seven years of plenty to avoid disaster in the seven years of famine, because of Joseph's wise advice (Genesis 41). We need wisdom to navigate life from a higher perspective, so we are not caught in avoidable problems, and I believe there is no wisdom greater than divine wisdom, which we can all ask for (James 1). We can sometimes get so comfortable when things are going well that we forget that the power and praise we are enjoying today might not be there tomorrow. Some people become so arrogant and wasteful in top, well-paying jobs that they cannot face life if that were all to be taken away from them. If they had made more effort to be nice to those who were not as privileged, and learned to live below their means while investing and caring for those in need, they just might have been able to get back on their feet when things changed. Living like that also helps us to keep the right perspective that money/position is not everything. The joy we get from giving and helping others is priceless. When we realise that the power and significance we enjoy is not a reason to look down on others, we can enjoy life even when those positions are gone.

It is very difficult not to get sucked in and defined by our roles, which is why I am so grateful to have an identity which supersedes any position I could ever hold in life. As a redeemed and loved daughter of God, it does not matter whether I am a GP partner or a cleaner at the surgery, Prime Minister or factory worker. I treat people well and hold my head high wherever I find myself. Humility is not about thinking less of yourself but thinking about yourself less. Not "everyone is talking about me". There is a bigger world out there that does not revolve around me. When I realise that my success is all part of God's greater plan, I do not consider it something to be arrogant about, because He can easily replace me with someone who will do His will in that position. This is a very humbling thought. The Owner of life can decide to move my station or even call me to heaven if I am not fulfilling His purpose for me where He has placed me. I do not live in fear that God might strike me dead or make me poor if I do not please Him, because I know that He loves me and is merciful. The Bible tells me that God's favour lasts a lifetime and His mercies are new every morning. I please Him because I love Him and want to be His "good and faithful servant" wherever He takes me. As children of God, we do not live in fear that we might fall from grace to grass because we know that the path of the righteous shines brighter and brighter unto a perfect day (Proverbs 4:18), and we appreciate every season of life. I love how the Apostle Paul put it - *"I know what it is to be in need, and I know what it is to have plenty. I have learned the secret of being content in any and every situation, whether well-fed or hungry, whether living in plenty or in want. I can do all this through Him who gives me strength."* (Philippians 4:12-13)

The excitement of getting that dream job, pay rise or promotion can sometimes make us forget the need to keep improving ourselves. Finally having the babies, friends or spouse we prayed for, getting that dream house or even the life-changing business deal should not make us forget the good principles and prayers that got us there. The blessings should not become an excuse to forget the Giver and His Word. We must continue to be diligent, humble and wise even when the privileges roll in. The influence, security and/or significance that come with success should not be a reason to forget that things can change. I know that some people find change more difficult than others and can struggle to initiate or plan for change, but winning in this game of life will require us to improve our attitude toward change because we know that it will always happen. Even the most successful people, according to worldly standards, have to retire one day as age creeps up and abilities fade. Contracts can end, jobs can go, health may fail, funding can be withdrawn and children will grow/change. It can be an exciting or depressing time, depending on how we lived during the high-flying years and the state of our hearts. If we focused only on the success or power when things were going well, there would be nothing left when it is gone. The unseen kindness and eternal investments will always be there for those who are wise. Change is still hard even for those who plan and live well, but we can be sure that they will come through better if they do not give up.

Servant of all

If I am being honest, the idea of being the "servant of all" does not sit well with me, especially as I have no problem being waited upon. I know this because I have lived for 14 years with a man who genuinely has the gift of service and would cater for everyone's needs before his. When we were dating, my husband would wash the dishes at my house or help in the kitchen when I was cooking. I could tell he was not just trying to impress me, he really liked helping. Even though he only knew how to make one or two dishes then, he would always make a proper meal for us when I visited. Now he is the MasterChef at our house - whenever he finds time to cook. At church, he was always on his feet setting up, serving others and packing away after the meeting. His job as a community pharmacist fitted perfectly with his nature because he loved serving customers, even when he had junior staff available to do so. His servant's heart is so large that he would deny himself good things to be able to give to others. I am so pleased that God gave me a husband like this so that over the years, we have rubbed off on each other to grow and find a good balance.

Being the servant of all does not mean letting people walk all over you. It is an intentional bowing low to honour others. It comes naturally for some, but it is definitely a work of the Holy Spirit in my life when I serve others. Naturally, I could easily attend an event and leave without lifting a finger to help, while my husband sees everything that needs doing at the venue and often ends up helping the organisers on the day. My mind generally expects that people have a plan to sort out their own responsibilities and will sort it, or ask me for help if they need it. Living with my husband and life experience has helped me to appreciate that people might not have it sorted and they might not want to ask for help. It has been great to work as a team where my husband can see a need and I can suggest better ways to help without enabling irresponsibility/laziness or overstepping boundaries. By God's grace, I can now also see and act on issues I would not have noticed before. When we are confident in our identity and motives, we do not need to worry about humility making others think less of us. My bending down to clean up vomit does not make me less of a doctor. If Jesus washed His disciples' feet, who am I to be too proud to help anyone? I love that my medical career and charity work give me many opportunities to serve others, not just in church or at home. Jesus said that whoever wants to be the greatest in His kingdom must be the servant of all. When we serve, we show people God's love in practical ways. People might forget what we said or did, but they rarely forget how we made them feel. Service looks different in different scenarios. We have heard of civil servants and servant leaders - they are serving just as much as the waiters and butlers.

God has blessed me with the ability and confidence to do all I do, so I consider these to be types of service - as well as caring for my family and friends. People might misunderstand our motives and even criticise us for doing what we feel passionate about. They might complain that you are too keen or naive, too open or vulnerable, too generous or people-pleasing. They might even take offence at *how* you did or said something, overlooking the main point and what was achieved. We might get angry or dejected when people do not appreciate our service, but I just want to end this chapter by encouraging us to look past their comments and focus on keeping our peace. We talked about how our peace is our power. When we allow flippant comments about the good things we do to get to us, we might become unproductive and just as bitter as some of the idle people who make them. There are times when we carry on as if we are not hurt, but it is important to check ourselves to ensure that we are not letting their poor understanding of us affect our view of ourselves and the power we have to change the world. Keep improving yourself and continue serving however you were designed to, for therein lies greatness.

CHAPTER 3
The Power of Yesterday

Learning from mistakes

My father used to love reminding my siblings and me of this Bible verse when we were growing up, "*People ruin their lives by their own foolishness and then are angry at the Lord*" (Proverbs 19:3) I have understood it better with time. Sadly, it is still true today that people get angry at God for things in their lives that are consequences of their own decisions or even the wider sinful state of the world. Instead of learning from our mistakes and moving forward, we can get stuck in cycles asking "Why me?". God is All-powerful but He gives humans free will. He does not force His ways on us. We have to choose to follow Him if we want to enjoy the benefits of His wisdom. In His amazing wisdom, He can direct our lives for victory, even when there are still people around us who choose to ignore Him. I am so glad that I am not God because the thought of juggling the balance of power and allowing free will in a world you created sounds stressful to me. Imagine allowing your children to do whatever they want from when they are born, in a house you own, while knowing that you are big enough to stop them and wise enough to see the terrible consequences of some actions they might choose. Not many of us can take it for a week. Yet, God allows us to live life however we want, even if it means ignoring His Word, and then we get angry at Him when things go wrong.

My children watched a movie called "Yes Day" where the parents allowed the children to have or do whatever they wanted on that set day, and they kept asking us to have a "Yes Day" too. As much as I want to believe that my children know their parents well and have some sense after almost ten years on earth, I would still struggle to agree to a "Yes Day" now. Even with adult children, parents still find that they need to offer guidance from time to time, but the dynamics are different then. However, we hope that if we have done a good parenting job, they can live a "Yes life" as adults because we know that they are making mostly sensible decisions. It is the same reason that the Bible says we can have whatever we ask for, according to God's will. The more we know God and His will, we start to pray according to His will and live a "Yes life". His Holy Spirit helps us to think like Christ and prioritise what He does. Having money, comfort and avoiding pain become less important than growing spiritually and showing people God's love. We will make mistakes as we go through life, but we learn from our mistakes without giving them the power to control our future.

Learning from our mistakes will usually need reflection to understand why things went wrong and what we could have been done better. I have learned that it sometimes takes a change of perspective to see why things went wrong and avoid future mistakes. If you have the same mindset that got you into the situation in the first place, you will most likely be thinking in the same way still when you come across a similar situation and react in the same way. Disaster sometimes happens to open our eyes to the error of our ways, even if it is all we have known from childhood. Instead of beating ourselves up about our mistakes or "blindness", we can accept the forgiveness that God offers, forgive ourselves too and make restitution where possible. People have hurt others terribly in the name of religion, business or culture, only to find out years later that their whole thinking was wrong. Jesus did not come to bring religion but a loving relationship with God and salvation for all. The Apostle Paul went on to do great things as a man of God after God opened his eyes and stopped him from killing more Christians. The mistakes of our past only have power over us and our future when we refuse to let go. It is like driving in reverse through life when we keep letting issues of the past hold us back. There might be people around us who make it their business to keep reminding or punishing us, but they can only have the power to affect our future if we let them take away our peace and focus. Most success stories include episodes of failure and regret, but the people who win are those who choose to focus on the possibilities of the future, turn the bad experience into a stepping stone and move up to better things. Taking back the power from events of our past will help us to face the future more confidently.

Changed for life

There are some things from our past that change us forever. We see people struggle for years due to childhood trauma and experiences that damage their self-esteem and personality, but there are also people who have been changed positively for life because of experiences they had in their early years that gave them a great sense of identity, self-worth and resilience. I remember my uncle used to call me "doctor" even before I got into medical school because he believed in my dream. My father used to tell me how intelligent I am and my mother showed it by how hard she worked to make sure that I went to the best schools, even after my father lost his job. There were discouraging comments from some relatives and friends, which I chose to ignore in order to stay focused and strong for the journey ahead. The negative comments I heard cannot be compared to the trauma of abuse that some people experience in childhood, but I have seen people who have been able to overcome possible lifelong damage by choosing to be "powerful not pitiful" through faith in Jesus.

Even as someone with a relatively good childhood, I have seen how some of the experiences of my past can still affect me today, but I have to choose which of those changes I can live with and which I have to purposefully unlearn. Undoing such significant effects of past experiences can be a painful journey but will be worth it when we know the kind of future we want. It is a shame when I meet people who genuinely believe that they are too old to change, and I generally am not close to such people because I like to surround myself with people who are getting better and helping me to do the same. Psychologists use all sorts of theories and techniques to help people process and deal with unhelpful thoughts or behaviours, and I do encourage people to get psychotherapy when needed, but I have found that improvement starts with a decision to not let the past have that power over my present and future. There is too much at stake to let my or someone else's unhelpful comments or actions ruin the rest of my life. I sincerely hope that other people also do not spend the rest of their lives in misery because of anything I said or did. Most of the issues we blame for our unhealthy behaviours would have been from the first thirty years of our lives. Is it worth being miserable for the remaining 70 years, assuming we are lucky enough to reach 100? Even ten years of life is too much to waste because of past experiences and mistakes.

I realised that experiences of lack in my past have made me uncomfortable around the topic of money. Writing my book, *Money and Mental Wellbeing*, was a great opportunity to process my thoughts and help others too. Now I have to consciously remind myself that people are not trying to annoy or trigger me when we discuss money, but I have allowed myself to continue with some of the thrifty habits I learned in those days because it is always easier to spend more than it will be to cut down if you get used to an expensive lifestyle that you cannot afford long term. I also have to be careful to not pass on unnecessary limits to my children, who are blessed to have more than I did as a child. My parents did the best they could with what they had, and it is also my responsibility to do the best I can for my children with what I have. With more knowledge/power comes more responsibility. I have to lay aside any negative issues from my past, consider the knowledge and resources at my disposal, and prepare my children to succeed in a different world from what I saw growing up. We sometimes focus so much on passing on money and wealth without paying attention to the life skills and spiritual health that money cannot buy. I am grateful that I had a rich childhood in terms of faith and love, so I choose to focus on that as the life-changing power of the past to hold on to.

Age with grace

I think the reason why I am excited about turning 40 is the realisation that I have been blessed with many yesterdays, or many Christmases, as they say. When I was growing up, if people wanted to joke about someone looking young for their age, they would say that the person has seen many Christmases. In a society where women want to feel young and pretty, people might be tempted to hide their age or try to pass for younger. I am so blessed to have many older friends who have aged well, not just in appearance but also in accomplishments, so I genuinely look forward to getting older. It is a terrifying thought when old age is seen as a time of irrelevance and boredom, but that is not the kind of old age I wish or plan for. Our impressions of grandparents and elderly people from our past can influence our thoughts about ageing, making it a thing of dread rather than gratitude. I often remind my patients, who complain about bony wear and tear issues of old age, that "Getting old is a privilege denied to many".

We are not sure how long we will live but we know how long we have already had. There is power to be drawn from the experience we have gained over time. One of my friends used to tell me how he is now "gliding on his experience" in a top position at work. He was enjoying being able to sort issues easily

when I was giving them the benefit of the doubt, I will not stoop so low as to waste my time planning revenge. The Bible says that it is like heaping burning coals on someone's head when we are kind to them despite their hypocrisy and bad intentions. I choose to see the situation as an opportunity to show them God's mercy because they probably have issues I am not aware of. Even people we hold in high esteem have flaws and will get things wrong sometimes. I may be upset when someone annoys me but I do not hold on to it in a way that affects my perspective of my past. I surely do not then generalise to say that the experience was all bad. Focusing on positive thoughts releases feel-good hormones which are good for my intellect, mental and physical health. Most of the antidepressants we offer patients to treat anxiety and depression work by increasing the availability of serotonin, which the body can have more of naturally when we avoid toxic negative thought patterns. Philippians 4:8 tells us to fix our thoughts on what is "*true and honourable, and right, and pure, and lovely, and admirable. Think about things that are excellent and worthy of praise.*"

Sometimes "bad" things happen that are no one's fault. It might just be a change of season or an unusual twist in the journey of life. I remember feeling like the rug had been pulled out from under me when a writing contract I had years ago ended suddenly, and I was not sure if I would be able to find something else to replace the income. It was a contract I really liked because it gave me the opportunity to write freely and get paid for it. It felt like free money because I enjoy writing, but most companies will not have a budget to keep paying writers indefinitely. The company contact was polite and explained the company's new plans, which made me feel better because I was not just being replaced. I look back on those days and am grateful for the time it continued for, instead of being angry that it ended. I am grateful for the experience and contacts I made through that job. The money was just what we needed for that season of life before I became a qualified GP with higher earning power. Even if they replaced me with someone else, the right perspective would still be to thank God for the period for which I had it and look forward to what next God had for me. I have since taken on many more exciting roles, building on that experience and using skills I learned from there. I could allow that experience of suddenly losing a contract to make me paranoid and reluctant to accept future offers, but the right perspective of that memory allows me to still go for opportunities - with better safety netting.

There is so much strength we can get from remembering all the challenges we overcame and the "huge" problems that did not eventually crush us. When I need money now, instead of remembering the days when we struggled to pay my university fees in tears, I remember that God who provided such huge sums of money then can do it again in His own time - and He always does. When I lose a job or contract now, I am partly excited because I have seen that God sometimes clears away the good stuff to make way for better. When I pray for a sick loved one these days, I trust that God who healed me and many before can do it again; and if He does not, I know that He will give us the strength to face the situation. Selling houses these days does not come with the worry I used to have around finding a buyer fast, because I know that God works in His own perfect timing, which is always for my good. Psalm 23 tells us that we have all we need with God as our shepherd, so whatever I do not have now, I do not need now. God has proven Himself over and over again in my life, so I choose to trust Him even when I do not fully understand everything that happened in the past. I recently got irritated about having to change cheap batteries frequently in clocks and toothbrushes at my house, before I decided to not be cheap and just buy some better quality batteries that will last. The batteries made me think of how we keep using the same fallible energy sources for the journey of life, when we have access to God's supernatural strength to do life better through Jesus. He is the firm foundation and solid rock for life in every season. I was so touched by this lovely old "Weaver's poem" that a wonderful Christian neighbour in her 80s told me about:

"*My life is but a weaving between my God and me. I cannot choose the colours, He weaveth steadily. Oft' times He weaveth sorrow; and I in foolish pride forget He sees the upper and I the underside. Not 'til the loom is silent and the shuttles cease to fly, will God unroll the canvas and reveal the reason why. The dark threads are as needful in the weaver's skilful hand, as the threads of gold and silver in the pattern He has planned. He knows, He loves, He cares; nothing this truth can dim. He gives the very best to those who leave the choice to Him.*" - Grant Colfax Tullar

History on repeat

For us to live extraordinary lives, we need to take advantage of the privilege of hindsight and do what we can to prevent negative history from repeating itself with us. I love hearing stories of people who came from difficult backgrounds to create a beautiful life, completely opposite to what they experienced growing up, against all odds. It is easy to give up and think that we have no choice if something is the norm in our family - but there is always a choice. I did not have to study in Nigeria because most people in my family did. I did not have to become a Christian because my parents are. I also did not have to go to university because my father did. I looked at the consequences of their choices and decided if that was what I wanted for myself. I looked at the pros and cons to make decisions for my own life. My children may decide to look at my life as a doctor/author and decide to go into different professions, or not go to university at all. They are more likely to want to become professionals like their parents because it is usually easier to stick with what we know as children, but when we become adults, history and upbringing cannot continue to be the excuse that we use for how we live, especially if it is not working.

I am grateful for the good things my family taught and showed me, but it is my choice today whether to continue on that path or try something different. When I look back through generations in my family, I see mostly hardworking and honest people, but also some obesity and alcoholism. It would be unwise of me to choose the wrong path with this knowledge, as well as all the additional information we have from science, but I understand that everyone's journey is different. Science teaches us that some things have a genetic element, which we cannot change, but we can do our best to mitigate any risks to our well-being. We also know that nurture not nature is sometimes responsible for what we see running in families. If we eat the same foods and have the same attitude to exercise, it is very likely that we will all end up obese. If we struggle with poverty and frustration due to limited progress in life, we might end up turning to alcohol. I should be much more vigilant about even the simple choices when it comes to obesity, work and alcohol, because of the power of hindsight from the knowledge of my family history.

The effort we put into breaking the cycle of abuse, poverty, alcoholism, teenage pregnancy, depression, crime or whatever negative thing we find in our wider family's past will help to make life better for future generations, not just ours. A Nigerian preacher used to say, "If you come from a poor family, do not let a poor family come out of you". Poverty is not just about money, some people are poor in virtue, faith and relationships. History is known to repeat itself, so it will not be the end of the world if you end up just like your parents or relatives. It might even be a good thing to be just like them if they lived well. Utilising the power of yesterday makes me want to do better than those who went before me, to use their success as a stepping stone to do better, so that my children have more to aspire to. I do not want an ordinary life that only fits in with what everyone expects. I want to be all that God created me to be. That can sometimes be difficult to imagine by only looking at the history of my family. Some of us have dreams and goals that might be firsts for our families or even countries. History is full of people who did great things even though they did not fit in with the popular thinking of their time. We can look back at history to learn and make better choices, but also use the power of that knowledge to build a better future, instead of letting it limit us.

Knowledge is power

I have found that ignorance is really not bliss, as they say, because the consequences of ignorance can sometimes be more painful than the knowledge of unpleasant facts. We cannot continue to use ignorance as an excuse, if we want more from life, especially now that there is so much information online. I know that access to the internet may be a challenge for some, but where there is a will, there is a way. I used to have to borrow books from my kind friends, which they might have borrowed from the library themselves, to be able to prepare for exams when my library access was blocked for late payment of tuition fees. I would keep studying in faith praying that my fees would eventually be paid so that I could take the exams and complete my degree. If I waited till my fees were paid and library access was sorted, I would have paid dearly for wasting time on worry instead of preparing in faith. It took a lot of mental strength to do that, which I know came from God, but I would not have made the effort to study in those sad times if I was not aware of the looming exams and the consequences of failure. It would have been very disappointing to fail my exams after my family stressed so much to pay the school fees eventually. It was my responsibility to pursue the information I was missing from lectures I was banned from because I did not want to suffer even more with resits. I could have been angry at God for not providing the fees "on time" every year so I could have a smooth ride like other students, but knowing that God owns the whole earth and still allowed me to experience that makes me consider that He had a greater plan which was not all about my comfort. There is so much I learned in those days that a degree course does not teach.

We say what we do not know does not hurt us, forgetting that lack of knowledge could be hurting us in a worse way. I ended up having to study Anatomy as my first degree at 18 because I did not know that most UK applicants showed evidence of healthcare-related work experience on their medical school applications to be considered serious about wanting to become doctors. I focused on getting good grades and was shocked to be rejected by all the medical schools I applied to. I was then advised to get another degree while getting some work experience, which cost me three years of fees and study. As someone who likes to look back with the right perspective, I am grateful for the positives that came out from that time, especially because I met my husband during my first degree, but I can also see that having the right information might have made my journey easier. No one else in my small college went on to study medicine and I did not know any British doctors, but I could have made more effort to find one for advice if I knew the power that the knowledge would have given me in the application process. We can also look back at other people's journeys to gain knowledge that will help us in the future. This is why I enjoy watching or reading biographies - with my children, and sharing my story with others.

One of my favourite lessons from my early days in psychiatry is that a good predictor of future behaviour is past behaviour. It can take effort to get to know people and their journey through life up to the point where we meet them, but that knowledge is power if we are considering having a meaningful relationship with them. I am amazed when people decide to get married and are proud to say that they do not care about each other's past, because "love is all that matters". When such people start having inevitable serious marital problems, they dig up information from their past and realise they would have avoided that relationship if they knew how that person had behaved in the past. The consequences of their ignorance might even include mental health problems for their children who have been traumatised from watching that relationship and its breakdown. Even in the areas of work and business, we do ourselves a favour to fully assess the pros and cons before making commitments. We might get carried away by an advert offering a huge salary and perks, without caring about the details of the job, how much time we would end up spending at work and the risks involved. I am not against taking risks, but "to be forewarned is to be forearmed". We cannot always have every relevant piece of information at the start, but we can dig for what we feel we need to know when making decisions instead of just making excuses for ignorance. We can retrain for skills we lack, read books and ask experts, instead of muddling along blindly with limited information. I am not very good at keeping up with the news, but I surround myself with knowledgeable people to make up for that, because there is also power in community.

Consequences

We are living now in the consequences of choices we or others made in the past. That is how much power yesterday can have over today. As we cannot change the past, we can review it and gain knowledge to help us create a better tomorrow. It is a free world and we can make our own choices, but sadly, we do not get to choose the consequences. If we choose to live just to satisfy our desires and pleasures, we will need to prepare for the consequences which can be very unpleasant in future. Galatians 6:8 says, "*Those who live only to satisfy their own sinful nature will harvest decay and death from that sinful nature. But those who live to please the Spirit will harvest everlasting life from the Spirit.*" This is a deep spiritual truth that some might struggle to accept, but I have seen unfold in the lives of people around the world. If we want to live extraordinary lives, we need to follow the life manual given by our Creator. We reap what we sow - choices have consequences, even for people who pray! Throughout the Bible, we see examples of people who laid down their natural desires (and fears) to please God and gained everlasting joy and blessings for generations to come, while others rebelled and suffered curses for themselves and their families.

The consequences of our actions can have far-reaching effects, even into the next generation. We ourselves might still be enjoying the rewards and blessings from the prayers and good deeds of a relative from years ago. I have heard of grandchildren finding faith in God years later because of the prayers of their grandmother. There are also families still struggling with shame and pain from choices that a deceased relative made years ago. Some family names can get you into places, while some keep you out. I see the blessings and favour of God upon countries that have godly principles because of decisions made by their forefathers. God is merciful - Jesus died and rose again to make a way for us to receive forgiveness whenever we decide to turn away from living according to our sinful nature. Instead of taking God's mercy for granted, we can learn from what has happened so far in our families and countries, and choose to make better choices going forward, so that future generations will thank us.

We can build on the good choices made by those before us and put a stop to the negative things that have been passed down. When I was growing up, my mother owned a restaurant and there was always food at home. She would sometimes cater for large events and bring leftovers home. She also donated pastries for church events, so there was plenty of opportunity for my sweet tooth to be kept happy. Everyone loved my mother's baking, and I grew up seeing plus-size women in my family and church. I used to get lovingly teased for being too skinny, because being overweight was seen as a sign of good living in those days. My grandfather was also a big tall man who enjoyed sweets. I have no idea if they even diagnosed diabetes there then. My grandmother died at the age of 68, and it was interesting to see that a lot of the thinner, poorer people in their village lived very long. Looking back now with medical knowledge, I can see that there might be an obesity gene in the family, but lifestyle choices are definitely a big contributor to the problem. It is my choice now to either make changes or carry on with the traditions of what we know now to be unhealthy eating habits. My grandfather was also a respected teacher who adopted and trained many children. The high value placed on education in my family is something I want to pass on to my children, but we need to make changes to our eating habits, which are sometimes not easy to maintain. I am sure that my grandfather, who eventually lived to around 100 years, would be so proud to see what a good education has helped me to achieve, but he would be even happier to see that we are going further than where he got to with the limitations of his time. I am also proud of my mother who did not consider herself too old to change and has intentionally lost so much weight in the past few years with a healthier lifestyle. Reversing well established mindsets, habits and their consequences is not easy, and I must applaud everyone trying to do this - wherever you are on the journey.

Lasting impact

It is great to be able to enjoy the benefits of the hard work and good choices of people before us, but we also need to be thinking about the impact we are having because today will soon be the yesterday that others look back on. Having a sound mind and peace is not just so we can have comfort and die without problems, we ought also to leave a lasting impact on the world around us. We will not all do big things like Billy Graham or Barack Obama, but we can make a difference in our families, workplaces, professions and neighbourhoods. As a newly married woman in 2010, there were many issues my husband and I discussed because of the interesting nature of our marriage. Even though both our families are Nigerians and Christians, there were major cultural differences because we come from very different parts of Nigeria. We decided early in our marriage to build our home on principles of the Bible - not based on his Yoruba culture or my Bajju culture. We chose to pick the good aspects of Nigerian and British culture that we and the Bible agree with and leave out the rest, so we can have a happy home. I have seen marriages break down or suffer because the wife or husband insisted on doing whatever their parents did, without even understanding why it was done that way in those days.

Our parents are human too and would have made choices based on the information and resources available to them. It would be a shame for us to make the same mistakes they made, despite having more information and hopefully spiritual maturity, by building on what they taught us. I believe that the changes we brought about in our extended families as a young couple will make life easier for the following generations who will not have to deal with some unnecessary conversations and stressful expectations. One of my friends reminds me of this too whenever I try to impose my personal preferences on my child - "Is it a sin? Are you the same person as your mum? Is your daughter hurting herself/anyone with her action/choice/preference?" If the answers are all no, we can find ways to accommodate different personalities while pleasing God, instead of creating mountains out of molehills. We can sometimes destroy our opportunities to have a long-lasting impact and influence when we focus on irrelevant or material things and destroy important relationships. Romans 12:18 tells us, "*If possible, as far it depends on you, live peaceably with all.*" We may need to have difficult conversations and make changes to find that place of peace. Sometimes we agree to disagree, but we should not accept situations that leave us without peace and power to flourish as God intended.

As we try daily to make a positive impact on the world around us while making history, we need to remember that success is not static. Just because you got fit after three months at the gym does not mean that you will be fit for life. It takes continuous work to maintain that physical fitness in the same way that we need to keep learning and improving ourselves to remain relevant and strong. That takes discipline and humility. I have had to regularly review how we work at Forte Charity for Inspiration over the past 15 years and accept help from several people for us to still be standing. The work did not finish after the charity launch and first fundraising event and project.

Making a lasting impact is not a quick job - it takes time. I invest time in my spiritual health through regular meetings with like-minded believers, hearing the word of God and praying always. I do not need to be in a certain position or place to communicate with God. I do not go to church, read my Bible or pray to make God love me more or to avoid punishment, because I know that God's love for us is a gift that we cannot earn through good works or rituals. The disciplines we are encouraged to have as Jesus's disciples are for our spiritual growth if we want the best that God has for us. Romans 5:8 says, "*God demonstrates His own love toward us, in that while we were still sinners, Christ died for us*." Surely there is no bad or good deed I can do now that would make God love me more or less. This gives self-worth and confidence for a joyful life. Living things usually grow or die, and growth is a journey that carries on until we leave this earth, but we know that our journey is not meant to be a lonely one, which is why we connect with others. "We rise by lifting others" and those little drops will make an ocean eventually. 1 Corinthians 15:58 encourages us in our faith to "*stand firm and don't be shaken. Always keep busy working for the Lord. You know that everything you do for Him is worthwhile.*" Having purpose, meaning and hope gives us strength for each day.

CHAPTER 4

Praise As a Hindrance

Preventing authenticity

If we are doing the right things, we will eventually get the praise and recognition our work deserves. Sadly, if care is not taken, the compliments and recognition soon become the motive for our actions and we end up missing our way. We might even start to do only what we think will bring more praise rather than what needs doing. As people chase the limelight, their inner light may become dimmer because they are moving further away from what they were created to be, sometimes to the point of making immoral compromises that dim their souls. The internal conflict from a guilty conscience, living a false life and constantly projecting a fake image can strain their mental health, which sometimes leads to physical health problems. It is a slippery slope when we let praise get to our heads and affect our reasoning. There is so much eye service in the workplace these days because people want to be seen, praised and promoted. I am sometimes amazed to see simple things like kindness and generosity being done for praise because business people have now realised that ruthlessness in business is no longer in vogue. Instead of becoming genuinely kind and caring, people make a show of it for the compliments they will get, especially now that we share everything on social media.

Although social media is great for raising awareness and making connections, it also makes it easier to see trends and follow what is popular. People who do not have a strong sense of identity can easily jump on whichever bandwagon is getting the most likes and comments so that they can feel good. It does feel good to be praised and liked, but that should not be the aim of life. Many great people were hated for doing the right thing because people at the time did not appreciate their wisdom. A lot of the freedoms we enjoy today were fought for by people who remained true to their convictions, even against popular culture. We can easily lose our focus and authenticity when we allow praise to be the motive for what we do. People may abandon a good project because the initial work did not get much praise, and follow trends for something less in line with their vision just so that they can get applause. So many writers today are also writing what they think people *want* to hear, and consistently ignoring the still small voice telling them what people *need* to hear. The world needs more authentic people who are not easily blown by the wind, but that boldness comes from sound spiritual health.

When I first started fundraising for Forte Charity for Inspiration, there were so many sceptics who felt that charity work in Africa was mostly a scam tactic. I remember one business owner told me that she was tired of seeing charities that are "here today and gone tomorrow" after taking people's money.

Not many 25-year-old international students were setting up charities to help people like them in Africa. I am grateful for the close friends and family members who supported us at the start so that I could continue with the vision even though there were no awards for us then. I could have joined a bigger established charity and ignored the vision in me to create a small charity that gets money directly to those in need without huge administrative costs and middlemen, and there is nothing wrong with joining an established organisation. In fact, I support many, but I would have lived a life of regret if I did not pursue the unique vision I had for Forte Charity, which I sometimes still feel pressured to change. So many unseen students and families in Nigeria, Ivory Coast and Sudan have been beneficiaries of the grants from our generous donors, and Forte is still going strong 15 years later with plans to reach more African countries. I am proud of the fact that our administrative costs are still less than 1% of our yearly budget, so that almost all the money raised goes directly to those who really need it. I have learned to be true to myself and my vision, even if we have to restrategize from time to time.

Difficult conversations

Most of us enjoy getting compliments and praise, especially for our work. It makes us feel good and valued. Sometimes it gives us the energy boost to keep going. As parents, we have learned to "catch our children doing the right thing" and give specific praise for that in the moment. This reinforces good behaviour and keeps relationships happy. No one wants to be told off all the time. Unfortunately, there are times when we all need to hear a bitter truth or hard correction. It is never pleasant, especially when we know that we have really messed up. We do not want to become a society so focused on feelings and praise that we cannot tell people when things are not going well, especially if it is for their own good. In British culture especially, we struggle to have honest conversations to say how we really feel when there is a problem. We give correction sandwiched with lots of praise and compliments, which might dilute the message, leaving the hearer confused about what is expected of them. I have had conversations where someone is really not happy about the way I work, for example, and tried to say it so fluffily that I had to go back and figure out for myself what they meant. Even as someone who has lived in the UK for over 20 years, it is sometimes difficult to decipher such conversations, no matter how well-meaning. I have sometimes had to decode such talks for international medical graduates who struggle even more with such communication during their training years in the UK.

It is a good thing to be aware of people's feelings and be generous with compliments, but it is important to retain the skill of clear communication when we need to say something less pleasant. Some people thrive on the "nice person" reputation that they struggle even as leaders to bring correction to people because they can only give praise and compliments. They are happy because everyone is their friend, but true friendship needs to be honest also. Even as a joyful, positive person, I try to be clear about how I feel about situations so that I am not just pretending to be happy. I remember having a conversation with a manager at a previous job where he asked after a few months if I had any issues to discuss. I told him that I did not have any issues because I like to keep short accounts and everyone in the surgery knows when I am happy or upset about anything. That was an exaggeration, but I do like to be open and honest. I told them from the start how I liked to have the same office to work from every day and made sure that the secretaries also understood how I managed my medical paperwork. Some doctors like to dictate, but I type my own letters, which I think they find helpful. Compromises had to be made - I had to accept the smallest office in the building because that was the only one available every day, but I was happy with that. We talked through the manager's expectations about my working hours and agreed on what I could commit to based on my childcare commitments and other interests. The compromise there was less pay for fewer hours, but I did not mind. It was a surgery that many doctors had told me would be horrible to work at, but I enjoyed my time there because I did not let praise and "positivity" stop me from speaking my mind whenever issues arose.

I have seen people become so good at praising others that they genuinely cannot have the conversation when correction is needed. They simmer in their annoyance and keep showering praises on the colleague even with a big elephant in the room. They might ask someone else to tell the person what they really want to highlight or start showing it by their actions in ways that are unhelpful for the relationship. When we realise that being a positive person who is generous with compliments does not have to be a reputation, we can be free to be ourselves and say how we feel. People are more likely to take our compliments more seriously and respect our views this way. I like to think that I can be positive but truthful. Sometimes we choose to overlook wrongs or give people more time, but we should not let the need to praise people stop us from being authentic in our relationships and workplaces.

No news is good news

When we become so dependent on compliments and praise to appreciate our own work, we can become dejected if no one is noticing. So many podcasters stop podcasting after just a few months because no one is sending them praise or comments. People get depressed and more desperate when their social media content is not getting the clicks and likes they expected. This desperation might drive people to seek attention online by posting unhelpful content or sexually provocative dressing, for example. That only ends up attracting the wrong attention or attention from the wrong type of people. I remember years ago when someone tried to tell me about sharing other types of content and "buying followers" so that my social media account would look impressive. He laughed when I said that I was not interested in such gimmicks because I wanted to reach real people with an authentic message. I have been doing my Happiness Over Stress podcast for over a year now and I know that it is making a difference to people's lives, even though it is not No. 1 on Spotify or getting 100,000 likes on social media. The real compliment for me is when I meet someone who might never comment online but tells me in person or by private email how much my podcast encourages and inspires them.

We have to learn to understand that no comment can also be a good thing. In my line of work, that is surely the case, because most of the people who read or listen to my message are busy and hardworking. They might not have time to write comments every time they find something helpful. There are people who follow me silently and might even find it hard to admit that they are learning anything from someone like me. I do not do it for the praise, I would rather they get the help they need from my books or podcasts in the privacy of their homes, and make better life choices than continue in ways that are detrimental to their mental health. When it comes to medical work, we commonly tend to hear back from patients only if they are worse or no better, so no news is usually good news. Rarely, patients will kindly send in a Thank You card and flowers, or even write a good review for our surgery. Children are taught to say "Thank you" but a genuine show of appreciation from family members does not happen every day. Your child might not be getting weekly awards in school or compliments from teachers, but that does not mean that you are a bad parent. Most schools only call a parent during the day when something has gone wrong, so no news is good news there. We also do not always hear or see how much our children are improving because of all we do for them. The benefits of good parenting can take years to show. We cannot function well if we are always chasing praise and compliments to reassure us.

We can learn to give ourselves a pat on our own backs after judging our work honestly. Sometimes, formal recognition or compliments will come and give us a great boost, but we cannot give up before then. It could also be that we are not yet at the high level we are aiming for, so it is important to keep working hard to get there. The Bible tells us in Romans 12:3, "*...Don't think you are better than you really are. Be honest in your evaluation of yourselves, measuring yourselves by the faith God has given us.*" We have already talked about humility and there are several books on managing imposter syndrome, so I just want to end this section by saying that we should not let the absence of praise for our work right now stop us from appreciating how far we have come and pressing on to greater things.

What will people say?

People like to associate with visible success. They will compliment you on getting a nice house, fancy car or big promotion, but you hardly ever hear anyone saying well done for choosing to spend sensibly, taking on less debt or prioritising family time over money. They might say well done for going out of your way to help someone but not well done for setting boundaries and looking after yourself so you can last longer. You need to give yourself a pat on the back for those decisions because they sometimes do not look glamorous or worthy of praise. Only you know how well you are really doing, so do not get distracted by weightless compliments and praise if there is really no progress. People can get caught in a trap when they enjoy the praise for a big promotion or massive house, and can no longer cope with the responsibility or payments. They might get caught up in other people's expectations for help they got praised for offering, which is now too stressful to continue. They would rather live stressed and consider every option, except stopping or "losing" the thing they were praised for. I remember watching a series about money where the woman had an expensive car, which was paid for by the pyramid scheme company she worked for - only if she kept up with high levels of sales. She was aware of the terms and how much she would have to fork out for it monthly after three months if her sales figures were to decline, but she chose to get the fancy sports car to appear to be moving up in life. When she started struggling to make sales, as can happen with any business, she could not imagine going back to driving a regular car because of the question that bothers most people these days, "What will people say?"

This makes one wonder whether we own stuff, or if it is the other way round that our stuff owns us. I love driving Mercedes cars, mainly because that is a car make that my father loves and I am used to them. I inherited the brand preference when my father used to joke that there are only two types of cars - Mercedes and others. There is nothing wrong with driving other cars, and I have to keep reminding myself that it is just a preference, especially when other people consider it a luxury car and assume certain things about you because of your car choice. As someone with poor parking skills, I usually drive a small hatchback with parking sensors, but I decided one day to be bold and get the bigger SUV I always wanted. I looked at many brands and buying options before I decided to buy a car that was not made by Mercedes as my first SUV. It was partly a cheaper choice in case I damaged it while getting used to parking a big car, but also to remind myself that Mercedes does not own me. I can confirm that I did not grow shorter or sicker by driving a less expensive car. I have heard financial experts say that the best car for you is the one you can afford to pay for with cash, not through debt. Life went on as normal and I am sure people did not spend time talking about my car - not the important people anyway. We can sometimes trap ourselves with expectations and financial burdens while worrying about maintaining the "look of success" when in reality success is not measured by stuff. Jesus said in Luke 12:15, "*Take care, and be on your guard against all covetousness, for one's life does not consist in the abundance of his possessions.*" and in Mark 8:36, "*For what will it profit a man if he gains the whole world, and loses his own soul?*" We can literally lose our souls and health when we focus more on getting more of the stuff we get praised for, than peace of mind.

This is not to say that we should not be ambitious or hard-working. I truly believe that my future will be better than my present, if I continue to trust God and make sensible choices, without worrying about what people will say or think. It does not matter if things look stagnant for a while, as long as we know where we are headed. David in the Bible was a shepherd boy and fugitive for years before he became King. Some people need to make big changes to pay off their debt so that they can make true wealth when they stop trying to impress others, while some just need to be content with what they have to be able to step into higher levels of success where they can be in a mental and financial position to truly help others. I remember feeling "poorer" as a new GP partner after making huge investments and tax payments in the first year of being self-employed. I was being congratulated for the partnership position, but I had to analyse for myself if it was really a promotion. It was definitely a good long-term career and financial move for me, but someone who may have copied me just to get the congrats, hoping to have more cash immediately to impress people would have been terribly disappointed. I might also be tempted to hold on to a partnership post that is no longer working out because of all the praise I got initially, but that would be a punishment for myself only. Thankfully, I am still enjoying the challenge of running a medical business, but navigating life from a higher perspective means that I would not stay somewhere that was no longer working for me just to keep up appearances or for past glory, because we sometimes have to let go of the good to get the great.

Satisfaction of a job well done

Giving compliments, thanks and praise is a good thing, but when we do something all the time, it becomes expected. It has to do with the concept of conditioning, where people learn that they get certain rewards for doing certain things. When it happens often enough, it becomes a shock to the system if we do not get the reward we were expecting. We use praise consistently in this way when training children or pets, but it can become a hindrance to good use of initiative and self-motivation when people become dependent on commendation to produce motivation. I believe this is the reason why so many adults struggle to do anything for themselves after they have left school. We pamper children with certificates for every little achievement, and people can even get an award for "trying". This makes the awards less valuable to those that really work hard and a thing of entitlement for those who do not. My children figured this out early in their education when they noticed that every child eventually got invited to an achievement assembly and even the naughtiest children sometimes got an award to encourage them to improve. Coming from a different time and country, I found it hard to explain this to my children, but have managed to pass on to them that we do well for ourselves, not just for the recognition. Jesus said, "*To whom much is given, much is required*" (Luke 12:48)

We are blessed with different strengths, gifts, knowledge, ability and resources. When we look at how others are performing as a yardstick for how much effort to put in, we are living by lower standards. If we only work hard when someone is watching, we are performing eye service. When we only do good if people are grateful, we deny ourselves greater rewards.

In workplaces, you might see staff who will only do well when there is a bonus or promotion connected to their performance. Organisations have these performance measures to ensure and reward productivity, but they can become a hindrance to people's ability to do good for the sake of the satisfaction of a job well done. I try to thank our staff regularly at work, but I prefer to make it meaningful and relevant rather than something expected for work they are already getting paid for. At home, my children will get thanks for running errands for me, but do not expect thanks, and certainly not money, for doing chores we consider to be their responsibility as people who live in the house. The least they can do is clean their own rooms and clean out their lunch boxes each day. I am even impressed when they come to thank me for giving their rooms a thorough clean at the end of the week or month.

Everyone works differently, but we can try to encourage an atmosphere where people are self-motivated and work to a standard they can be proud of, even if no one praises them. Writing this book very early on winter mornings before going to work is not something I am doing because of the money, fame or praise, but as something I can be proud of whether anyone appreciates it or not. I really hope that people will appreciate and be helped by it, but I would not want to be discouraged if it did not sell ten million copies or get millions of five-star reviews. I remember making small books as a child in Nigeria by stapling pieces of my writing together. My parents were supportive of my love for writing but they did not pay much attention to it at that age. In fact, I got more chores to do whenever I seemed to have too much time on my hands! Now, I see my daughter typing away on her computer, not caring if I have time to read and praise her work, because she loves it and enjoys the satisfaction of writing a good story - when she is not engrossed in a video game! We miss out on achieving so much when we let excessive praise or the lack of it hinder us from doing our best simply for the satisfaction of a job well done.

Lying to be nice

You can probably remember watching a talent show audition and wondering who allowed a terrible singer to come all that way to sing so badly on television. It ends up being comedy for all involved, except the humiliated singer who really has no idea why people outside their family are not praising their voice. It usually starts with a mother trying to be encouraging, then a father trying not to be the bad guy, then siblings who have been taught to "be quiet if you do not have something nice to say" and probably grandparents who do not want to be banned from visiting. People sometimes even add "white lies" when giving fake compliments, not realising that the person is being truly deceived by those comments. In trying to be nice, we can sometimes find ourselves turning into liars and deceivers, so our inappropriate praise becomes a hindrance to that person's self-realisation and growth, which is usually not the intention to begin with.

I do like the common saying from British mums telling children to be quiet if they do not have something nice to say, so that they do not say the very mean things they sometimes feel like saying when they are upset. I have said this to myself too, even as an adult, because words are powerful and cannot be revoked once spoken. It can take up to ten positive comments to repair the damage done by one negative comment, so we do need to be careful about what we say and how we say it. However, this should not be a reason for us to swing the other way and say things that are clearly false just to protect people's feelings. We might never really know how much weight our words carry until we see how our words have affected the confidence and choices of the listener. We can be honest and polite at the same time. The Bible says that "*Lying lips are an abomination to the Lord, but those who deal truthfully are His delight*" (Proverbs 12:22). Even if society has tolerance for some types of lies, whatever colour we might want to call them, we can choose to be people of integrity that say what we mean and mean what we say.

We have all said things or exaggerated at times without meaning to, and God is faithful to forgive us when we repent of our wrongdoing, but it needs to be a conscious decision for us to replace bad habits with good ones. It feels good to praise and compliment people but we can be doing them a bigger favour as friends by being honest to say when things are not so good. Proverbs 27:6 says that "*wounds from a sincere friend are better than many kisses from an enemy*". I have had friends who started avoiding me after I expressed concerns about a dangerous step they were about to take as Christians, but I prayed for them believing that God would direct them out of the mess whenever they were ready to listen. Pride prevents some people from speaking up when they realise their mistakes, so they suffer in silence, but I have been blessed to have people who came back to me years later saying that they should have listened and appreciated me as a friend or relative for speaking the truth to them even when it was not what they wanted to hear. It is never an easy position to be in, and I would just smile supportively if it was someone I did not know well, but love makes us speak the truth to one another when needed. Thank God for good friends in my life who do the same for me.

Silver linings and dark shades

I have learned over time that not everyone sees the silver lining in the clouds as easily as I do. I am not sure if it is mostly to do with my personality or the intentional spiritual growth from spending time in God's word over the years. I am convinced beyond doubt that God is in control of my life, everything happens for a reason. If God allows something, it will work out for my good and His glory. I can understand how life can be very worrying for someone who does not have this belief and trust in God. There is so much uncertainty around us, terrible news every day in the media and so much to be wary of as people find new ways to harm and scam fellow human beings. When I sit with people talking about everyday life, it can sometimes get depressing because they are focusing on the real and hopeless situations in the world today. It is even worse when we talk about the state of some African countries which has led to so many people migrating and living like slaves in other countries. There is no quick solution or obvious silver lining to share and we have to be honest about this. There will be things that we do not completely understand, so all I can do as a child of God is to pray about the things I cannot control and trust the One who can. I am then reminded of the fact that so many people are finding deeper relationships with God even amid the chaos and that is worth being grateful for - although, this might be difficult to understand from a non-Christian perspective.

The joy that we have in Christ cannot be shaken, even with all the evil going on in this world, but we need to remain sensitive and compassionate to those who do not share in this hope. We can listen and support in the best way we can, without letting them feel that our life of praise and joy makes us so "heavenly focused and earthly useless". We can share their tears and think of practical ways to help, because we know that "faith without works is dead". There is no use in me singing praise to my Jesus happily when the world around me is burning and I will not lift a finger to get water. Living from a higher perspective is knowing that we are "in this world but not of this world", and letting our light shine through the darkness. Darkness has never, and will never overcome light. We bring hope and peace wherever we go, not by ignoring real problems people are facing, but by sharing our hope and caring through action. We just need to be careful also not to get sucked into negativity and wrongdoing when we try to empathise or support.

It can be a difficult balance to stay joyful but approachable to those who feel hopeless; to stay faithful but open to those who choose to live by different standards. I think I have gotten better over the years in this area, and am still improving. When I was at university, a close friend told me years later that some of my female friends were pretending to have similar values around me because they knew I was a Christian - he knew things about them that were surprising to me. I was open about the fact that my boyfriend and I were choosing to live apart and save sex for marriage, even though it was not a popular way of doing things and we could have saved on rent by living together while dating. I was confident in sharing that we were only obeying God in that way and had nothing against anyone who chose to live differently, especially if they were not Christians. I had close friends who lived differently but I tried to stay focused on God's word for direction for my life so that I would not be influenced away for God's plan for me. It was difficult to keep our hands off each other as an engaged couple and there were many temptations, so it is only by God's grace that we waited until our wedding night. It is also only by God's grace that we stay faithful in marriage, because there is still temptation everywhere. My husband and I know that God would not love us any less if we have sex outside marriage and repent, but we just wanted to follow God's way and reap the rewards, which we now are. I feel that we are better able to trust each other in marriage and have enjoyed getting to know our bodies after the wedding without psychological complications, which sometimes come from sexual experiences of the past, whether good or bad. Some students said that they had to "test-drive a car before buying" and some even wanted to sleep with everyone they could before committing to one person. I believe that sexual intercourse is not just a physical activity, and looking after my spiritual health through a close relationship with God helped me to look after my mental and sexual health, even when my parents were not there to monitor me. I realise that it is their choice to open up or not when I speak with people, but I need to continue to show love and remain non-judgemental in my conversations, so that my success and confidence does not become a hindrance to them sharing their challenges or opinions.

One-hit wonder

As the Apostle Paul said, "*I have not yet reached my goal, and I am not perfect. But Christ has taken hold of me. So I keep on running and struggling to take hold of the prize. My friends, I don't feel I have already arrived. But I forget what is behind, and I struggle for what is ahead*" (Philippians 3:12-13) There is always room to grow in our spiritual journey. We are learning every day and keep pressing on for more. We cannot let the praises and success of yesterday stop us from achieving greater heights. When we take our eyes off the prize, like a runner looking backwards in a race, we will suffer loss. No matter how great the successes of yesterday, we can forget what is behind and press on for more if we do not want to become a "one-hit wonder". If we consider past successes as stepping stones for greater things, there is no limit to how far we will go in life.

I remember how we used to get class positions in school in Nigeria. The teacher would rank the whole class, based on their exam and test performances, from 1st position to last position. That was usually the first thing on your report card - 2nd out of 25, 1st out of 30 or 15th out of 20, for example. I was surprised to find out that children are not told this in UK primary schools, but I can understand how that might cause distress for children these days. In my time, it taught us resilience and healthy competition. When I got 1st position on my report card a few times in a row, my father started asking me to compare my grades from the last term to my grades from the current term to check if I was actually improving. That was an important life lesson. I was not encouraged to relax because I was comfortably in first position, I learned to compete with myself and not others, so that now I am really not so concerned about what everyone else is doing, but trying to make sure that I am improving for myself. As I got older and did not care about A grades anymore, I have learned to set targets for myself and measure myself according to my own ability - not according to what others expect, because only I know what other challenges I am dealing with and what is a good result *for me.* Of course, there are standards we have to meet in our workplaces, but I will not hold myself back from doing my best if it is a lower standard than I know I can achieve. I will also not be too hard on myself if I barely meet the target in an area that I personally struggle with.

I remember there was only a 40% pass mark in the first year of my BSc course and other students kept reminding me that the "first year did not count", so they partied all the time and planned to work hard in years 2 and 3 which mattered more. I knew that bad habits are hard to get rid off, so I started as I meant to continue, especially knowing that my time at university was costing my family a lot of money as a UK international student who also had to work during the weekends. There were people who talked about working smart, not hard; those who got 1st class degrees even after going to most university parties; and those who ended up in top positions even with a third class degree. Looking at them, you might not be aware that they have photographic memory for exams, well-connected families, huge inheritances or previous work experience in their fields. We need to each run our own race, and not let praise and successes of the past make us feel too proud or comfortable to press on for all that God has in store for us in life, work, career, ministry and family. It takes more to finish well, even after starting well.

CHAPTER 5
Praise As a Tool

Gratitude

As a medical student I used to listen to a song by William Murphy called "Praise is what I do". It used to bring tears to my eyes because I was dealing with so many financial challenges at the time, and hearing a song remind me of how I could praise God in good and bad times made me cry. I knew from the Bible that God wants us to give thanks in all things (1 Thessalonians 5:18) and I knew that God deserves my worship and praise even if He never did anything else for me, but it was sometimes so hard to sing those words. I would often stop when it came to the part that said, "I vow to praise You (God) through the good and the bad" because I did not want to make a promise I could not keep. I was committed to follow Jesus all my life and knew I would not compromise my faith to do anything contrary to God's will for me just to get more money or have an easier life, but I was not sure I could praise God every day while waiting for things to get better.

Anyone watching me might have thought I was torturing myself by listening to songs about a good God when I was facing overdue debts and possible deportation. My parents were also struggling financially and my close friends had helped me the best they could already. All I wanted was to be able to pay my tuition fees and focus on my medical studies like other students, but lack of money was such a huge problem. I would have to remind myself that I still had things to be grateful for. I was never homeless or without friends. My family was there for me emotionally, even when they did not have money to give me. My academic ability and sanity somehow stayed intact. The same song reminded me that we praise God to be close to Him because we owe it all to Him. I found that when I turned my attention to praising God for *who* He is to me, rather than worrying about *what* I wanted Him to do for me, I began to feel better and gain strength for each day. The need to look after my spiritual health made me worship even when I did not feel like it.

Giving thanks and praise in all things does not mean denying the reality of our situation, but choosing to focus on a greater reality. Even though I was a poor student, it did not make me less of a royal child of God. I could trust that He was working it all out to make me the empathetic doctor I am today. I started to find more things to be grateful for when I chose to sing praise to God. He saved my soul from eternal damnation and gave me the gifts of everlasting peace and joy that money cannot buy. Even if He did nothing else for me, I could not praise Him enough for the rest of my life. In African culture, you come into a king's court with praise and gain favour from him that way. Even a wicked king would give good gifts to one he is happy with, how much more our loving Father who delights in our praises. Faith helps us to believe even before we see the answers to our prayers, so we can continue to give thanks and praise in all seasons. The simple act of singing praise itself does wonders for our minds and bodies, helping us to face each day. We see in the Psalms how David loved praising God, and even King Saul used to ask for music from David, which "refreshed" his soul (1 Samuel 16).

Praising God is a way of showing our gratitude for life and all we have. When we genuinely give thanks we begin to feel more positive and worship flows more freely. I use praise as a tool to start my day right, focusing on God as the one who blessed me with another day and giving thanks for all He will do through and for me that day. I am so grateful for apps like Spotify where I can find any song I want, or just choose a worship playlist to start my day. It is even better when I sing along because the words in the songs have power as we speak them out loud. I say good things about myself and praise the God who helps me to serve others by His power. Living a life of praise and gratitude helps me to find favour (or "luck", as some might call it) even in the face of challenges so that I have even more to be thankful for as time goes on.

Better health

Most of the Christian praise and worship songs we sing today contain truths from God's word about our identity and His great promises to us. The psychological effect of hearing and speaking words of affirmation, reminding us that we are victorious, loved, accepted, redeemed and safe in Christ releases good hormones like dopamine that make us have better mental health. Listening to music itself has been shown to reduce anxiety, blood pressure and pain. Studies have shown that listening to music improves sleep, memory, alertness and mood. Playing music gives our brains a total workout, which is why I encourage my children to play musical instruments. I am very proud of the progress they have made with the violin, piano and drums at such young ages. Listening to music increases the release of feel-good hormones, which we can all do with, especially in the dark winter months.

I discovered this simple mental health hack years ago and it has helped me to stay well even when work is stressful. I will usually listen to music on my way to work to get my spirit calm and mind alert, ready for the day's work and conversations. I also listen to music instead of serious podcasts or news after work, so that I can be more relaxed by the time I see my family after a long day at work. Most of my music is worship music which focuses my mind on God and the bigger picture. I sometimes listen to pop music but will quickly switch off anything that sounds negative or unhelpful because I am very aware of how powerful words can be on the mind. People can struggle with anxiety and depression for years when they continue listening to music and words that are not good for their souls. A lot of popular songs these days talk about broken relationships, sadness, lust and materialism. It might be okay to listen to them once in a while, but when we listen to things like that all the time, it soon shapes our worldview and begins to make us feel low or anxious. I would rather hear and sing about how loved and blessed I am, and how good and great God is.

Our music choices as parents can also affect our children's mental health. I am always so pleased when I hear my children singing or humming songs about God's love and power, because they have been hearing those from my phone or car. They might play trending songs on YouTube or Alexa sometimes, but the majority of what they hear is uplifting music. Even though I do not play any musical instruments, we have become a musical family because we intentionally put things in place that are good for our spiritual and mental health. When we praise God, we show that we depend on His mercy and we see more of His favour. We do not only praise God in good times or on Sunday mornings, it needs to be a lifestyle for us to see the full benefit of it. Even on Sundays in church meetings, people might be tempted to just do the motions when they worship, but there is real freedom in praising God wholeheartedly. His joy overflows from us to our homes and we can rejoice even in the presence of challenges. That overflowing joy also leads to praise and compliments for those around us too, which we know releases feel-good hormones to make them feel better as well. I love meeting up with other believers who understand the power of praise. We share songs that have powerful lyrics and help us to celebrate our God and the life He has given us.

Overflowing joy

Any situation we face can only crush us if we let it. Following Jesus does not mean that we won't have problems, but Jesus already said, "*I have told you these things, so that in Me you may have peace. In this world you will have trouble. But take heart! I have overcome the world.*" (John 16:33). Spirituality in Christ is not choosing an easy happy-clappy life. In fact, we will face mockery and even persecution when we stand firm in faith without compromise. We get through that by changing perspective, seeing things from God's viewpoint and celebrating like the victorious people He has made us to be. Romans 8 is my favourite Bible passage because it reminds us that "nothing can separate us from God's love" and we are "more than conquerors" in Christ, which is why you might see someone in a difficult situation finding the strength to smile and even help others. I remember Forte Charity for Inspiration was actually founded in 2008 when I was still trying to sort out my visa and tuition fees for medical school. When we praise God, we can trust that He is sorting things out for us, so we can go about doing what He wants. The overflowing joy that springs up from a heart of praise is so attractive that people want to be around you and you find even more favour wherever you go.

No one likes to stay around negative and complaining people. When people choose to complain instead of giving thanks and praise, they find that they end up even more lonely and dejected. There is a time and a place for therapy and sharing concerns, but we should not become people that constantly talk about our problems. Instead of magnifying the issues in my life, I choose to magnify God and trust that He is working it all out for my good. Even if someone actually meant bad for you, imagine the confusion for them when they see that you have remained joyful and strong through the trials. You just keep pressing on and being a blessing to others. As it was for Joseph in the Bible, the pit and prison that were meant for his destruction ended up leading him to his destiny as ruler of Egypt. When we live a life of praise, we try to see the best in people also. Forgive those who hurt you and enjoy true spiritual freedom. It is not possible to truly praise God and live a happy life when we hold grudges and refuse to forgive others.

Praising God helps me to see how small I really am and give Him the glory for all He has helped me to achieve, but it also shows me how great I am in Him. When people give me praise and compliments, I can accept them humbly, knowing that it is all by God's grace. In this fast-paced world, a commendation from one or two influential people might be all it takes to move you to the next level of your career. Instead of focusing so much on how to put in all hours at the office and get 100% on every test, I focus on serving the One who owns it all, and He leads my steps to the right places for promotion and favour. Prioritising God and time for worship has been something that has paid great dividends in my life, even when work was so busy and there were many people to impress. The time I spend in worship helps to refresh my soul and gives me perspective and solutions for the challenges ahead. I have experienced periods where God has helped me to be highly efficient so that I could still do all I needed to do for work, as well as all the other things I was meant to do, even after making time for church and prayer. Indeed, "the joy of the Lord is our strength" (Nehemiah 8:10).

You get what you expect

Have you ever noticed that people eventually get what they expect? Of course, this is a generalisation, but that is how faith works. We can be intentional to believe for good things or let our fear run wild with all sorts of possible disasters starting from our minds. The man, Job, in the Bible was a good man, but he experienced a terrible time of trial where he lost everything, including his children. One of his comments was, "What I always feared has happened to me." (Job 3:25). The main lesson from that story was that his faith did not waver, even in the tough times - he was later restored and rewarded abundantly. Job said during the tough times, "Though He (God) slay me, yet will I trust Him" (Job 13:15) When his wife and friends gave up, and even blamed him because they thought he might have been receiving punishment for wrong-doing, he stayed strong in faith and refused to "curse God and die", as his wife suggested. The Bible describes faith as the "substance of things hoped for, the evidence of things not seen" (Hebrews 11:1). People often say that they will believe it when they see it, but the higher perspective is to believe before you see, and that faith is what brings it to reality, which is why we praise God even before we physically see a manifestation of the answers to our prayers.

When we expect people around us to fail us, they usually do. We encourage people by telling them that we believe in them, hoping for the best and showing them their potential. People who constantly hear criticism and have low expectations placed on them will rarely succeed. Like a plant, when we nourish people with praise and good expectations, they flourish and rise to the occasion. When people receive compliments, it releases a feel-good hormone (dopamine) in the brain which is associated with pleasure, reward, motivation and positivity. It tells our brains to do it again and can feel just as good as a monetary reward. Giving compliments helps to affirm and reinforce positive behaviours at home and in the workplace, so it makes sense that we should be people who are consciously building others up with praise.

When we praise God, we are not doing it to make Him do what we want. We praise Him because He deserves it, but praise also changes us, as we learn to depend more on God as our glorious King. When we depend on the One who never fails, we cannot lose. The Bible talks about a wise man building his house on a rock, which was not blown away by the storms of life, but the foolish man builds his house on the sand and is left with nothing when the rain comes (Matthew 7). Jesus said that anyone who believes and obeys Him is building their life on solid rock. He has been my firm foundation and living hope. Whatever we choose to put our faith in should be able to stand the test of time. I am so sad to see such a rise in the rate of consultations this year for attempted suicide, because people feel so hopeless, even with so much money, technology, "friends" and pleasures. Praise is a tool that helps me refocus on the centre of my life, Jesus, who speaks to me through His word with guidance and hope for every day. Ignoring that important part of my life would only be a ticking time bomb to that empty feeling people eventually get without God.

Dance for joy

Instead of focusing so much on what is going wrong, we can choose to focus on God's promises and all He has already done. It can be tough with our minds wandering through the week's events, news headlines and upcoming bills, but I found that music is a great way to force my mind to have fun. Whether I am singing with friends/family or by myself, I feel so much better when I dance as well. God loves to see us praise Him with all we have got. Psalm 150:6 says "*Let everything that has breath praise the Lord*". We do not need qualifications, talent or music skills - just a thankful heart, which God fills with joy and overflowing blessings as we praise. There are times in my life when I refused to wallow in worry, praised God whenever I felt tempted to feel sorry for myself and looked back to see that God had sorted the issue in better ways than I would have. It would have been such a waste of my time to have been crippled with worry about something I could do nothing about. As I praise, I even get new ideas and strength to help others, so that the challenging time ends up producing something even better for the world around me.

Some might think it sounds crazy, but I have had situations where I did not even have the words to pray because the problem felt so big, but I sang praises to God instead, and miracles happened. My husband was admitted to hospital by ambulance one New Year's Eve. I was left with the children at home and had to cancel other plans we had for the week because I knew he would usually stay in hospital for at least one week with a sickle cell crisis. It happened to be a Sunday, so I decided to go to church with the children and praise God instead of worrying. My praise songs started from home because I honestly did not have words to pray and I trusted that God is in control. He had done it before and He will heal again. It was scary starting a new year that way, but I knew that God would help us overcome. Praise overflows from us in hard times when we fill ourselves up with the right things in the good times. Someone once described humans in trouble as a bottle being squashed with pressure. What bursts out is usually whatever the bottle contains, so I fill my heart with God's word and praise, so that my response in times of difficulty will be victorious praise and thanksgiving, which does not make sense to an ordinary person but has worked miracles for my life and mental health. Swearing, complaining, self-pity and anger do not seem like better options to me. We worshipped God joyfully without pretending that all was well, because I informed the church leaders. Friends in church prayed for my husband and he was discharged the next day! It was good to be able to dance and praise in faith even before I heard news from the hospital. I am so glad that I did not ruin my day or year because of that incident. I know that not everyone gets the answer to prayer that they expect, but total surrender to God means that even if He did not heal my husband, I would still praise Him, because He is Almighty God, not a genie that serves me.

Jesus said to his disciples in Luke 12:22-31, "*Therefore I tell you, do not worry about your life, what you will eat; or about your body, what you will wear. For life is more than food, and the body more than clothes. Consider the ravens: They do not sow or reap, they have no storeroom or barn; yet God feeds them. And how much more valuable you are than birds! Who of you by worrying can add a single hour to your life? Since you cannot do this very little thing, why do you worry about the rest? Consider how the wild flowers grow. They do not labour or spin. Yet I tell you, not even Solomon in all his splendour was dressed like one of these. If that is how God clothes the grass of the field, which is here today, and tomorrow is thrown into the fire, how much more will He clothe you—you of little faith! And do not set your heart on what you will eat or drink; do not worry about it. For the pagan world runs after all such things, and your Father knows that you need them. But seek His kingdom, and these things will be given to you as well.*"

Raise others

Even after years of reading the Bible and serving God, I still struggle with controlling my tongue and have to trust God daily to help me. These verses really challenge me to watch what I say: "*From the same mouth come blessing and cursing. These things should not be so, my brothers and sisters. A spring does not pour out fresh water and bitter water from the same opening, does it?*" (James 3:10-11) When we live a life of power and praise, it should also be a life of integrity. We cannot be comfortably praising God from the same mouth that we curse people, gossip and lie. These are all things that God's Holy Spirit in us helps us to leave behind, as we become more like Jesus our Lord. It is a lifelong journey, as our human desires continue to wrestle against our spiritual goals. Christ makes us extraordinary because we can do all things through him. Romans 12:2 tells us to "*let God change the way you think. Then you will know how to do everything that is good and pleasing to him.*" God does not override our free will so we need to submit to His power to change us. I have found that God often speaks to me during times of worship and praise through the song lyrics and Bible verses. He might speak to my heart through a preacher's talk or through a friend, telling me which way to go and where I need to change. Following Jesus is not all about feeling good and singing songs, there is a (sometimes painful) transformation that goes on as well in our lives, as we become more like Jesus in character. It takes discipline to stick with it but the benefits of spiritual disciplines have been found to lead to happier, longer lives. As we grow, we also support others to grow in their spiritual journey too. When people are down we stand with them and lift them up by praying with them and encouraging them through

God's word. The sense of community I have through church, with an atmosphere of praise to God has been great for my mental health.

Some people have found religious communities bad for their mental health when the core principles of love and service are lost. I do not think that every church is for everyone, and just because a church group does not suit your personality or circumstances does not mean that faith is bad. If they are allowing abuse and illegal activities in the name of religion, safeguarding concerns should be raised with appropriate authorities. When I was a student moving around, I always found a church family in every city I lived in, because I knew that having people around me with similar beliefs would help me to stay grounded and strong. Also because of Hebrews 10:25, which says that "*Some people have given up the habit of meeting for worship, but we must not do that. We should keep on encouraging each other, especially since you know that the day of the Lord's coming is getting closer*". We go to church not just for ourselves, but also to be there for others. Post-pandemic, people have struggled to get back into physical meetings and we are seeing the negative impact on mental health of this, even among Christians. Apart from the physical and mental benefits of meeting together regularly with others for encouragement, we build ourselves up spiritually in this way.

Churches will have different styles of worship and praise, some sing quiet hymns and some dance to contemporary music, but as long as they are doing things in love according to God's word, you just need to find where suits you best. God has all sorts of children so there are bound to be disagreements and mistakes from time to time, but with love and forgiveness, we can stick together and grow in faith. The Bible is full of advice for what to do when these things happen, and when we are humble enough to realise that we too are not perfect, we can find a church family to settle down with for the long haul. I have been so blessed to have been part of the same church with my family since before my husband and I got married. I am so happy to have had the privilege of watching my daughter make her own decision to follow Jesus and get baptised at the age of nine. Faith is a personal decision, and people do not automatically become Christians just because their parents are. As someone who has seen the great benefits of a life of faith in Jesus, I pray that all my family, for generations to come, will also find this treasure in their youth.

Watch your space

Another great aspect of faith that helps my mental health is being able to share it with my family. I am blessed to have a husband who also believes in Jesus. This was an intentional thing, when I obeyed God's word to not get into such an important lifelong relationship with someone who was not heading in the same spiritual direction. Having a man who also lives for Jesus means that we have fewer arguments and the same priorities. We make time to pray together as a family and teach our children about God, which creates a positive and powerful atmosphere in the home. The Bible has so much to say about the power of agreement and unity. When we have such an atmosphere at home, we are already winning in life. We manage the spiritual atmosphere of our home through prayer, praise and the power of God's word which we speak and read to each other regularly. We build each other up with praise, not just for what we are doing but for what we know God is doing in us by faith. This is especially important when raising children and helping each other to overcome our faults. People may not remember what we said but they usually remember how we made them feel. This is something I try to remind myself of when dealing with others. I have some relatives today who I hardly call because of how they made me feel as a child, and other people, who might not even be related to me, who I would gladly visit because it feels good to spend time with them. I do not hold grudges but am just not keen to be around or talk to negative people. When we maintain a peaceful atmosphere of praise and hope, people want to be around us, even though not everyone is meant to be part of our close inner circle.

It can be easy to fall into a pit of negativity and sadness, which then creates a downer atmosphere around our homes that people with spiritual discernment feel repelled by. We can use a habit of regular praise and thanksgiving as a tool to manage our atmosphere and reduce the chances of things getting stale around us. Worship is not just something that happens on a Sunday morning, it should be part of our daily lives. Our spirits feel quickened when we do what we were created to do. We honour our Maker and strengthen others around us. As we all have different schedules and commitments, we need to reflect regularly on how we are making time to look after our spiritual health. Just because someone goes to church every Sunday does not mean that they are strong spiritually. Spiritual health is about the relationship you have with yourself and your creator, which overflows into how you treat others. Online church services and private catch up with friends can be helpful when attending a larger meeting of believers is challenging, but I have found that I am stronger spiritually when I do those as well as the in-person church meetings. It is part of being intentional to manage my time and mental space in a way that helps me spiritually too. When we have important spiritual disciplines in our lives, we have less time for unimportant stuff that can be bad for our mental health. I genuinely do not have time to sit around gossiping or moaning after I have made time for church, Bible study, work, children's activities, couple time and personal reflection. Going to church is usually the thing that people drop off their diaries when things get busy, but that is not something I would encourage and we would need to think of how else we can feed our souls intentionally if we do that.

It can be unhelpful for our mental health to become too strict and rigid about church attendance and other spiritual disciplines, especially when it involves people who are younger in their faith journey. It can breed resentment, strife and guilt when people are made to feel as if God loves them less because they are not 'performing' up to expectations. Some churches even overburden members with several "mandatory" meetings and volunteering responsibilities, that they become so stressed managing that with work and family life. We do these things to build ourselves up, and there is freedom in Christ - people should be able to serve voluntarily and feel free to reduce church/volunteer commitments, if necessary. "The sabbath is made for man, not man for the sabbath" as Jesus said, but we should also be careful not to take God's grace for granted and only serve Him when convenient. King David said that he would not give God something that cost him nothing. When our time is so tight and precious, that is when we truly show our commitment to God by putting Him first in our diaries. We have seen popstars who start out great in church and drift away to drugs and depression when they get too busy with fame. Even when life gets busy, we can manage our spiritual space by regularly engaging in private prayer and praise. Even if you do not have Spotify or great musicians at your church, you can read the Psalms and sing from your heart to God. YouVersion is also a great Bible app that allows me to access God's word every day and anywhere on my phone. Thankfully, free Youtube is also well-stocked with edifying music, talks and movies that we can access to keep our minds focused on God at any time.

Count your blessings

Being thankful and singing praise comes more naturally for some than for others, but I cannot imagine anyone not being able to give thanks when they take a moment to actually count their blessings. No matter how poor or deprived you might think you are, there are many more in worse circumstances. When we realise that things can be worse, we can find something to be grateful for while giving our concerns to God in prayer. Singing praise is not a denial that life can be hard, but it helps us to refocus on the One who has all the answers. Even when we feel that He has not acted according to our expectations, we can trust Him when we remember that God is love and knows all things - we only see part of the picture. From a spiritual viewpoint, I feel so blessed that God opened my eyes to see my need for salvation, touched my heart to believe in Jesus and made me able to accept His gift of eternal life which gives me hope even in the face of trials. From a mental health perspective, I am so thankful that I can think clearly and cope with the daily stresses of life, I can make decisions and work as a doctor, while juggling other responsibilities as a wife, mother, charity trustee, school governor etc.

There are so many intelligent and much more qualified doctors who struggle to function due to poor mental health and cognitive decline, there are many intellectuals who struggle to believe in God and find the peace that I enjoy. Physically, I am so grateful for good health in my body, the ability to move independently, my senses working well and my body systems functioning as they should. I refuse to focus on any aches and pains, but to thank God for all the other parts of my body that work well. I am grateful for not completely damaging my knee while playing netball and for all the times God protected me from serious accidents and attacks. The Bible says that the wisdom of God's word is *"life to those who find them, and health to all their flesh"* (Proverbs 4) I am so grateful for all the times that God has healed me and my family from common colds and serious illnesses. People can develop serious complications from simple infections, but we often praise our good immunity forgetting that there are many others who had good immunity and died of sepsis. I cannot list everything I am grateful for, but I hope that this encourages you to give thanks and praise for your life too.

Our souls find strength and hope when we give thanks and praise for what God has already done and look forward to all He will do. Just as we *choose* to love and cleave in marriage for it to last a lifetime in spite of each other's faults, I realise it is also a choice to love and believe God, and that is the "narrow path" that not everyone finds. The Bible assures us that God is faithful to complete the good work He began in us (Philippians 1:6). We can grow in our trust in God when we remind ourselves of the great and wonderful ways He has already shown us His love. We can also overflow with joy and become people of gratitude in our homes and workplaces, leading to a better atmosphere and productivity. Gratitude has become a more popular mental health tip these days, and we need to be genuinely grateful for even the little things in life, especially when we realise that it is not because we are better or more deserving than anyone else that we have these things. In fact, some of the things God does not let us have are a blessing in disguise, for our own good. There are people who get rich quick and die young, while there are so many hardworking people around the world struggling in poverty and so many good people living in pain. So much does not make sense and we do not have answers to all the questions of life, but that will not stop me serving the One who does. I thank God for all the wonderful people I have met in the past 40 years and how God provided all our needs. I am so grateful to be blessed with such a great husband (Bolade) and two wonderful children. I thank God for hope and strength for times when He did not take away our troubles but helped us to overcome them. Even if everything changes, as long as I still have breath and faith, I choose to be grateful and praise God knowing that He is indeed working all things together for good for those who love Him.

Conclusion

I know that God is still working on my character and the best is yet to come, so I give thanks for all He will do too. I pray to never let the blessings that God has given me become a reason that I am too proud to worship Him. We are sometimes so busy with the things that God has given us - work, children, spouses, friends, hobbies, talents, houses, cars and businesses - that we forget to make time to spend with the Source of all things. I can only imagine how annoyed I would be if someone loved my gifts more than they cared about me, but God is so merciful and willing to accept us whenever we turn to Him. The only issue is that the Bible says our time on earth is limited, Jesus is coming back for those who have accepted His love and there will be no more opportunity to turn back to accept His forgiveness once that time is up. As someone who likes to plan in advance, I would rather make sure that this most important spiritual part of my life and eternal destination is sorted, even before investments, pension and retirement plans. Whatever people decide to do concerning their spiritual health and beliefs, it is important to be intentional rather than just burying our heads in the sand about this. Please, take time to check out useful resources to make up your own mind about your spirituality and mental health.

When I was coming to England on my own to study at the age of 16, my father reminded me of this Bible passage, which has really helped me: "*Trust in the Lord with all your heart and lean not on your own understanding; in all your ways submit to him, and he will make your paths straight.*" (Proverbs 3:5-6). Today, as one of the most educated members of my family, I remember to still trust in God, not my own ordinary human thinking or qualifications. I appreciate and use the knowledge learned from science and medicine daily, knowing that it is all part of God's wonderful nature and provision for us. Living a life of faith for over three decades with great results and several testimonies of God's faithfulness has made me conclude, like an experimenter would, that this is the best path for me to continue on for whatever years I have left in my life's journey. I have truly experienced joy in chaos and peace that makes no sense, as in the lyrics of one of my favourite songs, *Firm Foundation (He Won't)*, by Cody Carnes. It is such a blessing to sing this song with Christians worldwide who have also tasted this extraordinary life and are not just church-goers. I have discovered in my time and learning that Christ is the one who fills that God-shaped hole in our hearts, which qualifications, money, pleasures and selfishness cannot fill. It is too good not to share, which is why I hope that this book makes others explore their spirituality and find a life worth living.

It would be terribly selfish to keep such a treasure hidden when the world so obviously thirsts for meaning. We do not go around forcing religion down people's throats, but we can show them God's love by the way that we live. Even though there is no scientific evidence for a lot of spiritual concepts, many have discovered these truths by revelation, because God did not intend for spiritual matters to be evidenced in the same way that the human body is studied in anatomy classes. The emptiness our souls feel when we ignore spirituality is a strong indicator that there is more to life. The power of God cannot be denied, a life of praise cannot be held down. Jesus said to let our light shine that all may see and glorify our Father in heaven (Matthew 5:16). As we look after our physical and mental health, let us not forget to build up our spirits through staying in peace (which is our place of power), obeying God's word (if you believe) and praising God in all circumstances, which gives us joy and strength. **Power, Obedience and Praise (P.O.P.)** is how I plan to have a "popping" 40th year and beyond. Thank you so much for sharing in my reflections and I wish you wholeness in mind, spirit and body. **#popping40**

Questions for Personal Reflection

Below are some questions that doctors might use in a consultation, which might be helpful to reflect on after reading this book.

Adapted from the H.O.P.E. questionnaire

H - Sources of Hope

- What are your sources of hope, strength, comfort and peace?
- What do you hold on to during difficult times?
- What sustains you and keeps you going?

O - Organised religion

- Do you consider yourself part of an organised religion?
- How important is this to you?
- What aspects of your religion are helpful and not so helpful to you?

P: Personal spirituality/practices

- Do you have personal spiritual beliefs that are independent of organised religion? What are they?
- Do you believe in God? What kind of relationship do you have with God?
- What aspects of your spirituality or spiritual practices do you find most helpful to you personally (such as prayer, meditation, reading scripture, attending religious services, listening to music, hiking, communing with nature)?

E: Effects on medical care

- Has your current situation or state of health affected your ability to do the things that usually help you spiritually? (Or has it affected your relationship with God?)
- Are you worried about any conflicts between your beliefs and your medical situation/care/decisions? (such as dietary restrictions and use of blood products)
- Would it be helpful for you to speak to a doctor, clinical chaplain, community or spiritual leader?
- How do your beliefs affect the kind of medical care you would like towards the end of your life?

<u>Adapted from the F.A.I.T.H. assessment tool:</u>

F: Faith/spiritual beliefs

- Do you have any particular faith, religious or spiritual beliefs?
- What gives your life meaning?
- What helps you cope in times of stress or illness?

A: Application

- In what ways do you apply your faith in your daily life?
- Do you belong to a particular church or community?
- Is prayer or meditation important to you?

I: Influence/Importance of faith in life and health

- How do your faith and spiritual beliefs influence your life? Are they important to you?
- Has illness influenced your faith?
- Do your beliefs influence or affect your healthcare decisions?

T: Talk/Terminal events planning

- Do you have anyone you can trust to talk to about spiritual or religious issues?
- Do you have any specific requests/preferences if you were to become terminally ill? (e.g. terminal care options, living will or end of life requests.)
- Have you disclosed your wishes to anyone or your doctor?

H: Help

- Do you require assistance or help with prayer or faith practices? (Such as guidance, resources, facilities or accompaniment)
- Do you need to speak to a chaplain or religious leader?
- Are you able to discuss spiritual issues or your beliefs with your family, friends or doctor?

References and Resources:

- https://www.youversion.com/the-bible-app/
- https://alpha.org.uk/try-alpha
- https://www.biblegateway.com/
- https://dimensions.covwarkpt.nhs.uk/
- https://www.happymaps.co.uk/
- 'FAITH' ASSESSMENT TOOL: Neely, D. & Minford, E. (2009), FAITH: spiritual history-taking made easy. Clinical Teacher. 6: 181-185.
- Spirituality and medical practice: using the HOPE questions as a practical tool for spiritual assessment, G Anandarajah, E Hight
- https://www.rcpsych.ac.uk/members/special-interest-groups/spirituality
- Why spirituality matters in psychiatry, Dr Nick Hallett, 2016
- Spiritual care is stagnating in General Practice: the need to move towards an embedded model. British Journal of General Practice 2019 Jan; 69(678): 40–41.
- https://www.nhsgoldenjubilee.co.uk/application/files/6816/6936/7153/Spiritual_Care_Strategy_2023.pdf

Milton Keynes UK
Ingram Content Group UK Ltd.
UKHW021017130524
442628UK00016B/849

9 781739 741631